PURE LIVING

Mother Nature's Wellness

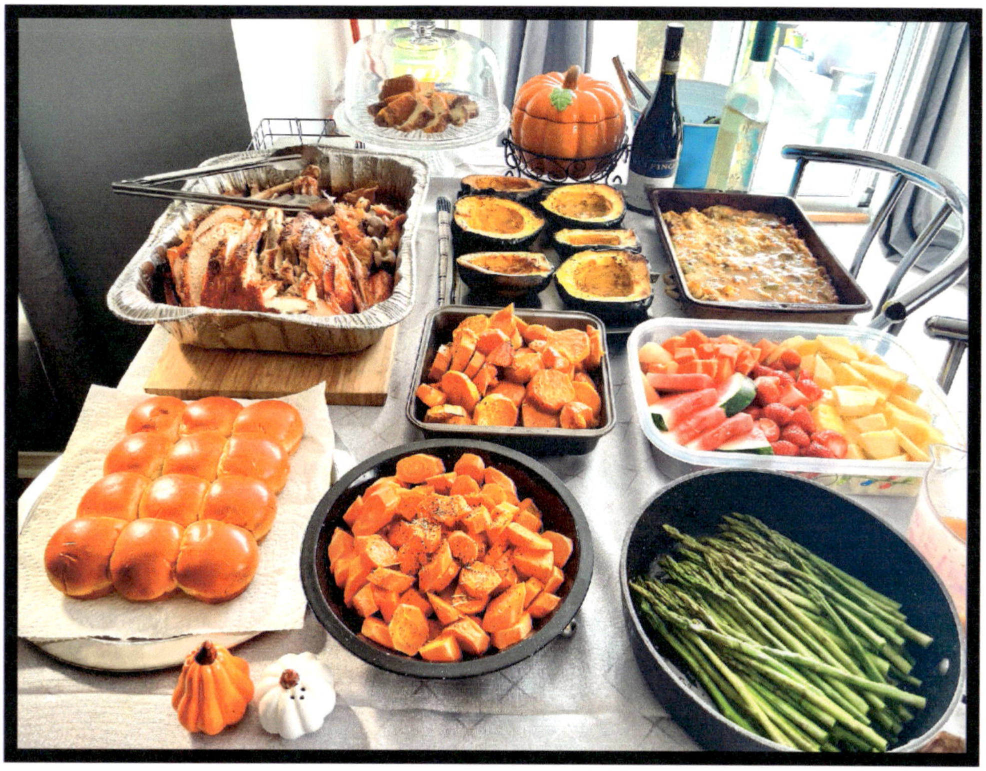

By

Michelle Ouderkirk

Dedication

I would like to dedicate this book to my family and my beautiful children.

Why I Wrote This Book

Step into a world where the countryside meets the magic of cooking. Picture a lovely house nestled amidst a breathtaking cornfield, where a young, eager learner embarks on a ***culinary adventure*** with their wise and talented grandmother.

Together, they unlock the ***secrets of homemade whipped cream***, a taste so extraordinary that even the finest store-bought pales in comparison. But that is not all!

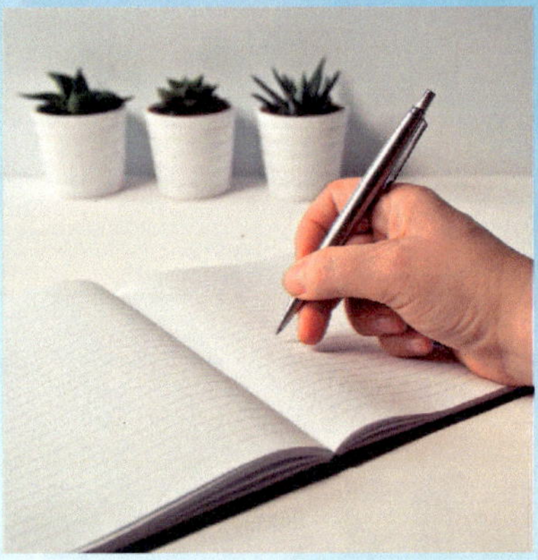

This whipped cream is not just meant for indulgence; it holds the key to a luxurious beauty ritual passed down through centuries. From bathing in milk like Kings and Queens to the wonders of the natural ingredients, join me as we journey through the kitchen of my beloved grandmother, a cook so skilled that even the kernels sought her expertise.

Get ready to immerse yourself in the wonders of food and discover the incredible products it can create.

Are you ready to be captivated by the enchantment of homemade delicacies and the secrets they hold? Take my hand on this journey together!

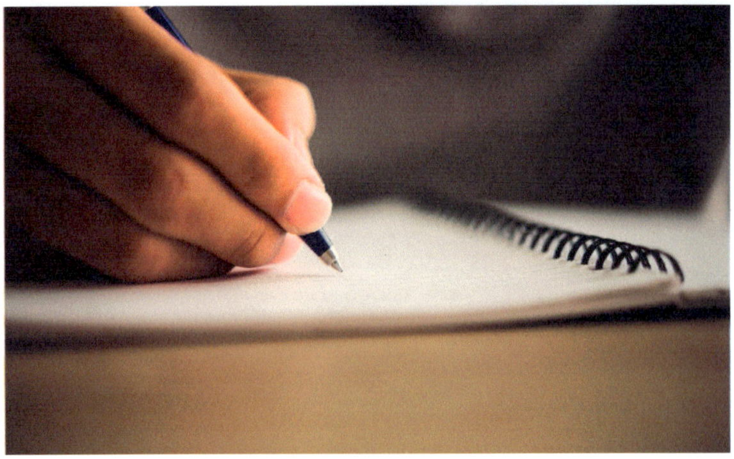

My Personal Skin Care

My personal skin care is simple, however. I apply all the factors, such as sleep, fasting, and natural whole foods, and have changed my indulgences, such as sugars, to better quality products that, in turn, do less damage to the body.

Because we all know that some sweets are just worth it, or we can just make better choices with the process things are made. Now, I want to discuss the benefits of whole foods and plant-based diets and the importance of consuming organic and locally grown sourced ingredients. I will include a shopping list and a few recipes to get you started.

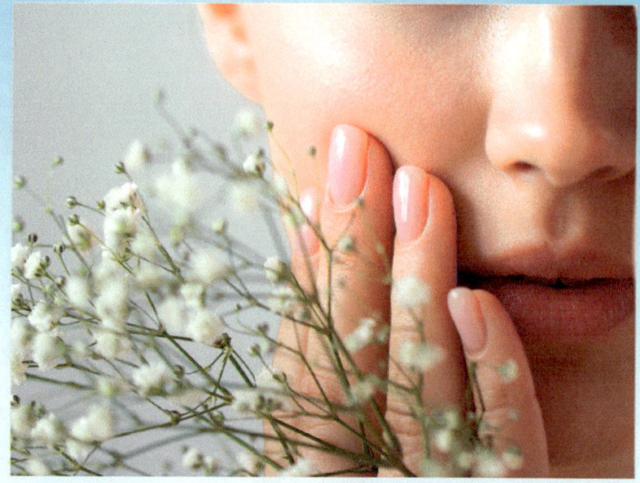

There is so much to cover. Let's go!

Jump right into natural products that can benefit overall health, starting with a focus on the face and skin. I use a few things now. Please understand that combining all the tips given will balance overall health, as natural products combined will only enhance your experience.

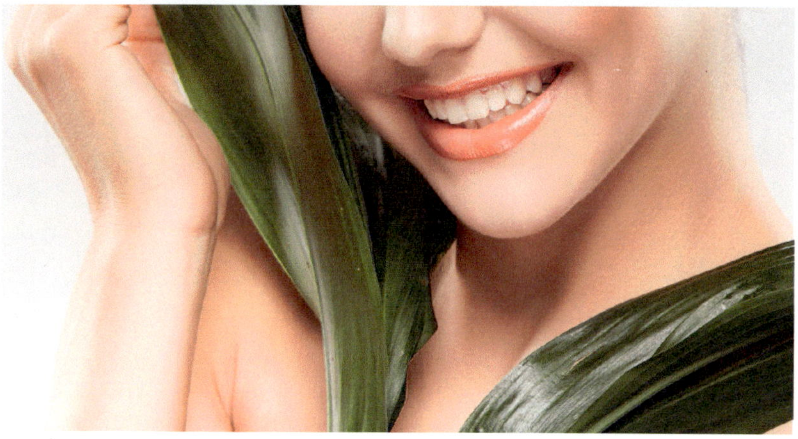

So back in my grandma's kitchen, we were making homemade whipped cream, still a family favorite – a simple, easy ingredient.

35% whipping cream; whip until fluffy!

In your bath, leave it on your skin for 15 minutes before washing it off, leaving the skin feeling soft and not tight. I usually triple the batch and fill my bathtub.

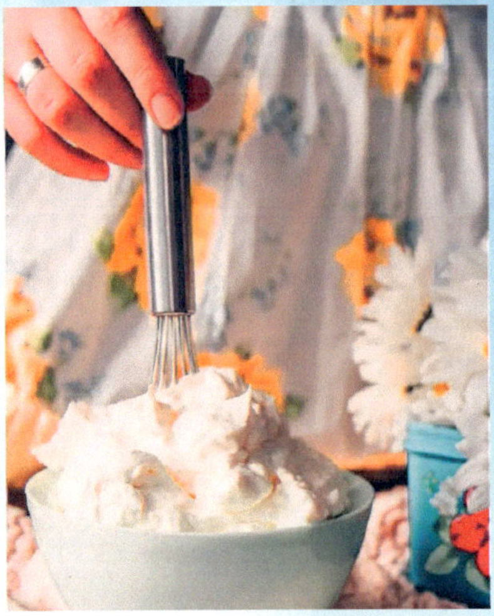

Listen, cream, whole milk, goat milk, lamb, and donkey milk have been used for years to improve skin, going all the way back to Cleopatra, along with kings and queens.

I am sure some of the things I mention might ring a bell, as many of us have heard stories of this growing up. I just happen to be that person that never stopped asking why.

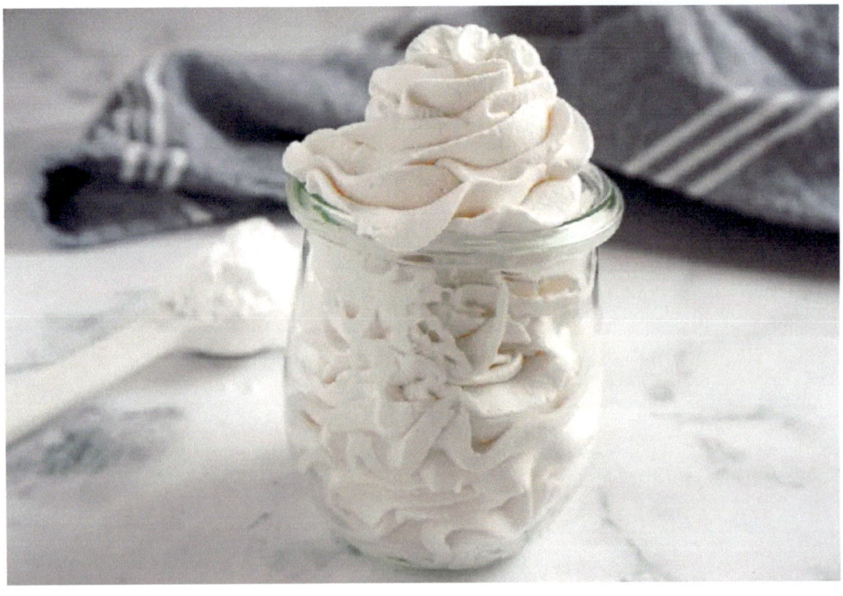

So, if you want to eat whipped cream instead, add a half cup of icing sugar after whipping along with 1ltr of whipping cream and a teaspoon of real vanilla, and your whipping cream is ready for use.

You can also drop one-inch-sized drops on a cookie sheet and bake for ten minutes by adding two whipped egg whites, which can be tinted for Christmas cookies.

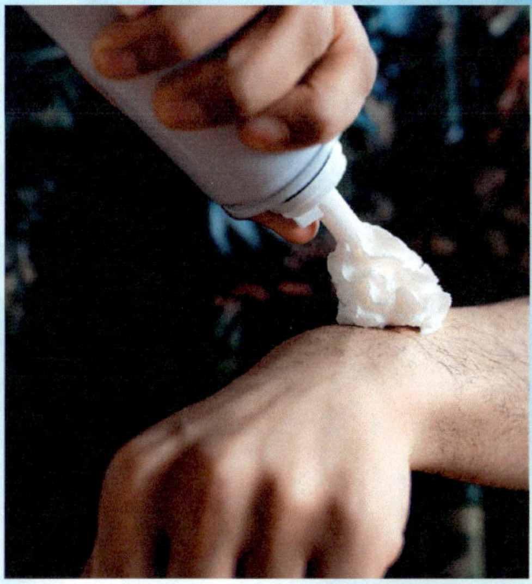

Some of you may have never heard of dairy products put on the skin, but they have a soothing, calming effect on delicate skin areas. Some may have heard of tallow, which is an animal fat that was used for many things, from skin softening to cooking.

But today, I am going to teach you about the benefits of using the proper oils and fats that can give you glowing skin and hair, so the following page will give you a list of fats oils that help the hair and skin maximize the benefits for you and get you headed on the right path towards optimal health.

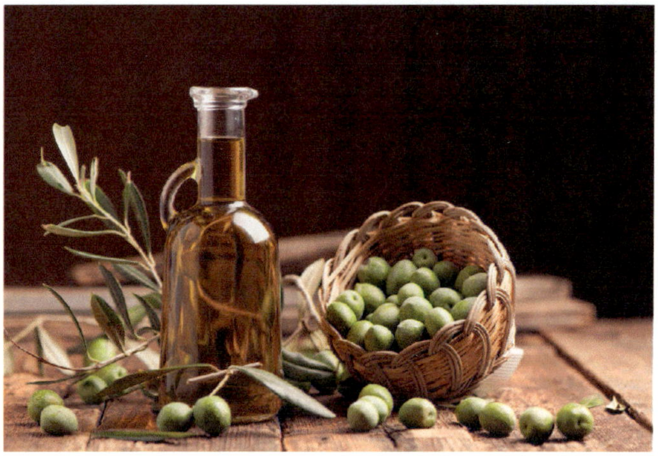

Keeping My Skin and Hair Healthy

I would like to include the fundamental principles of natural health, such as the importance of a balanced diet, regular exercise, stress management, and adequate sleep routine. I will provide some easily accessible and practical tips for implementing these principles to your daily life.

However, my personal skin care is simple. I apply all the factors, such as:

- Sleep
- fasting
- and natural whole foods

I have changed my indulgences, such as:

- Sugars, to better quality products that, in turn, do less damage to the body.

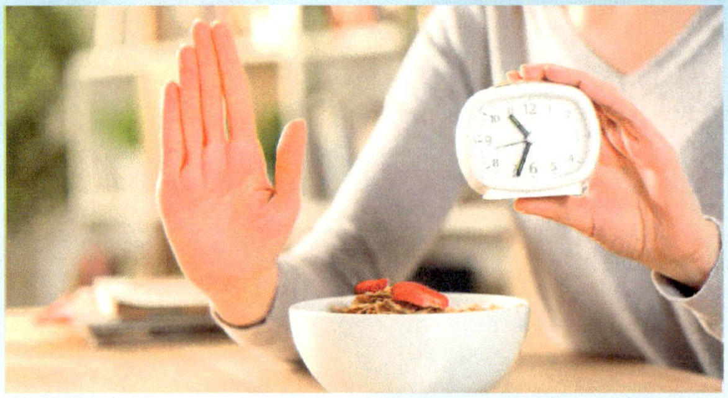

Now, I want to discuss the benefits of whole foods and plant-based diets and the importance of consuming organic and locally grown sourced ingredients. I will include a shopping list and a few recipes to get you started. There is so much to cover, so let's go!

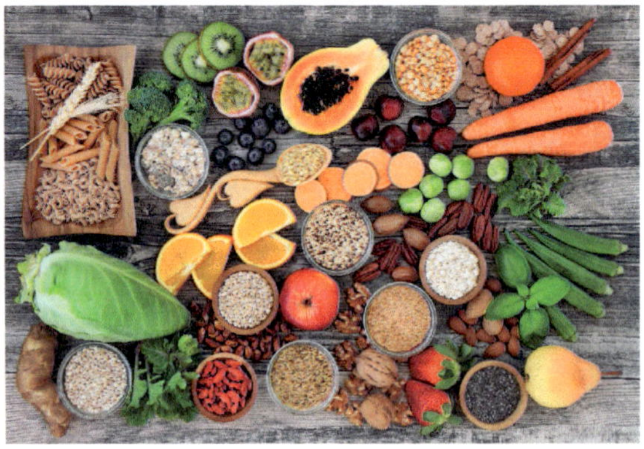

Taking Care

I have always had psoriasis, and when I was a teen, I started doing my research to get rid of this scaling skin on the back of my arms and neck that eventually moved to my ears. I was told you could try tar medicine or topical creams, but I was not satisfied with the chemicals or results. I started to study, and my results are fabulous, and I no longer suffer from embarrassment any longer.

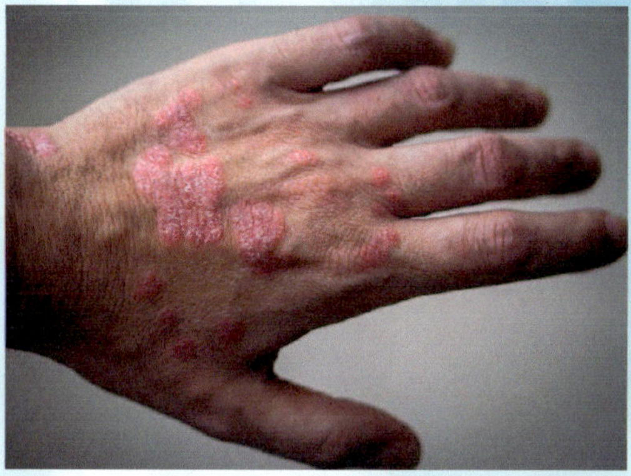

Using Sea Salt

Simply use sea salt in your baths. There is no fragrance, just natural salts like Celtic, Himalayan, or grey. In fact, I went so far later in life to add a saltwater pool to my home for the benefits, and it's great. So, along with my daily salt baths or swims, I only use two things on my body daily, which is my absolute favorite pear soap!

Here is a little cool information: it was the first soap ever made to sell as a bar of soap. The story is about two lovely farm ladies who entered a town fair competition by making this soap with all-natural farm ingredients and won.

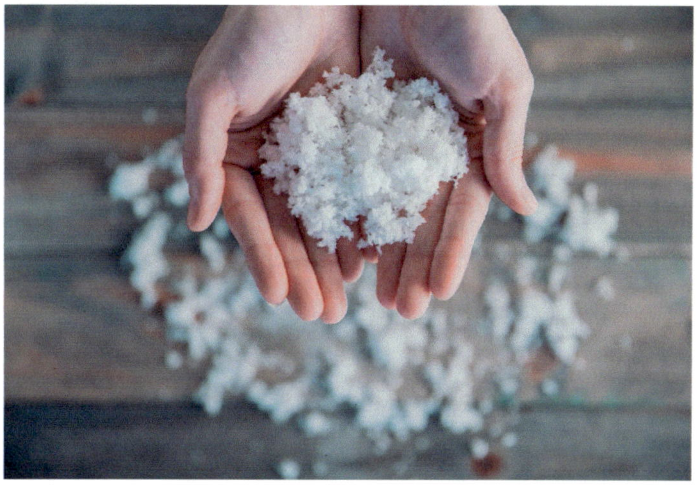

The Pear Soap

Now, if you are older like me, you will remember this soap. Pear soap is not actually a soap, as we are accustomed to seeing and using, because it does not contain detergents like its counterparts. The benefits of that are no drying of the skin and less chemicals left behind in your pores. I tell you that I cannot live without this Pear soap, which is an understatement; the way it clears acne and smooths and tightens the skin is incredible.

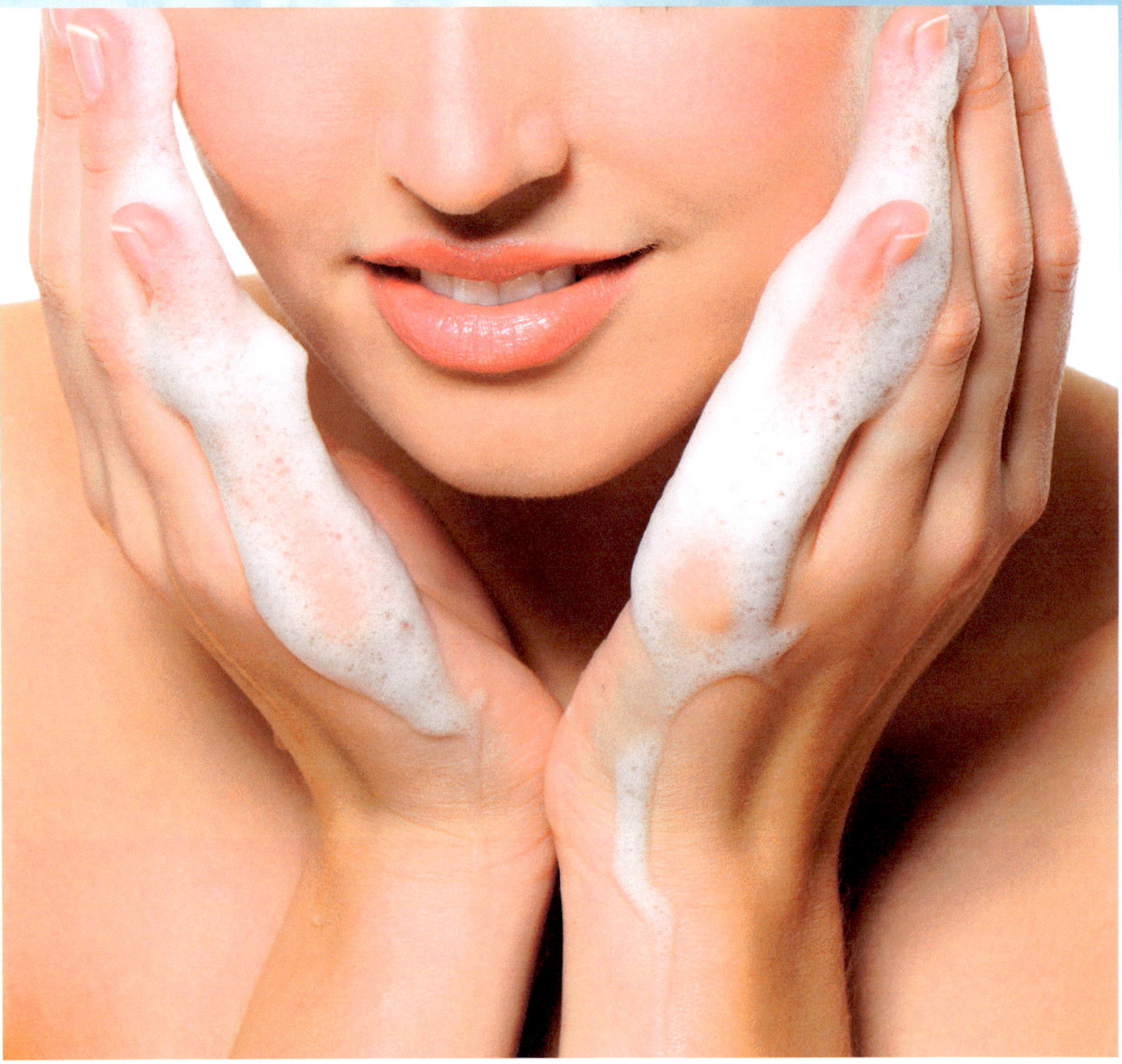

Unfortunately, they have changed the recipe over the years, and they sold the company. I have inquired with the original company about investing in or representing their product, but the new company never responded. I am, however, working on making my own soap closer to the original soap, so keep your eyes open for that. For now, I am still using the pear soap and it is the only soap my skin loves.

Moisturizing My Body

Now, for moisturizing, I use coconut oil and or olive oil mixed in a 1/1 ratio for the entire body, hair, and nails. Coconut oil on its own is fabulous for softening the skin and sealing in moisture.

But did you know that you can also take one teaspoon before bed for constipation, and you will not wake up running but instead feel relief?

Coconut can also be used for what is called pulling to brush your teeth with. It is the best oil to cook with because it has a high smoke point, which means it can withstand elevated temperatures without smoking or burning like olive oil.

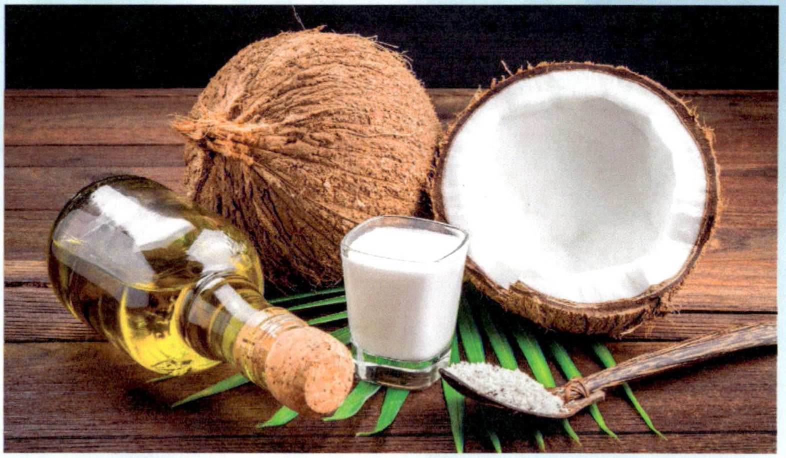

Toothcare

Speaking about teeth, stop wasting money on expensive whiteners that only strip the enamel of your teeth, weakening them. Baking soda can be used to clean your teeth to whiten once monthly with a teaspoon of each: peroxide, baking soda, and sprinkle of salt, and you will never use whiteners again. I also have included a recipe for homemade toothpaste in this book to make at home if you wish.

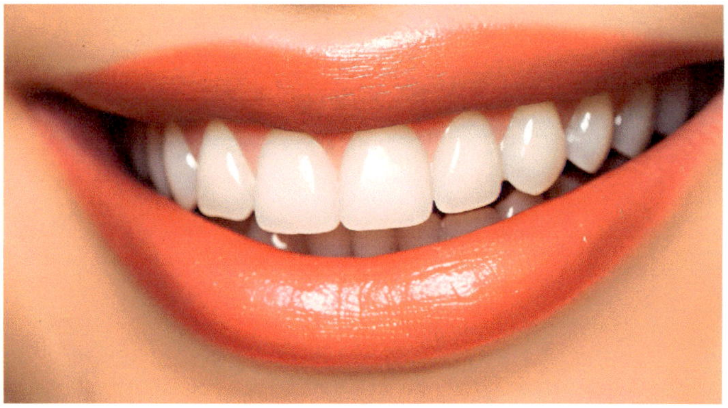

Hair Care

Let us talk about hair. Investing in a horse bristle brush is worth it, as it can hold the natural hair oils and help take healthy oils along the hair shaft, promoting better growth and strength with less breakage

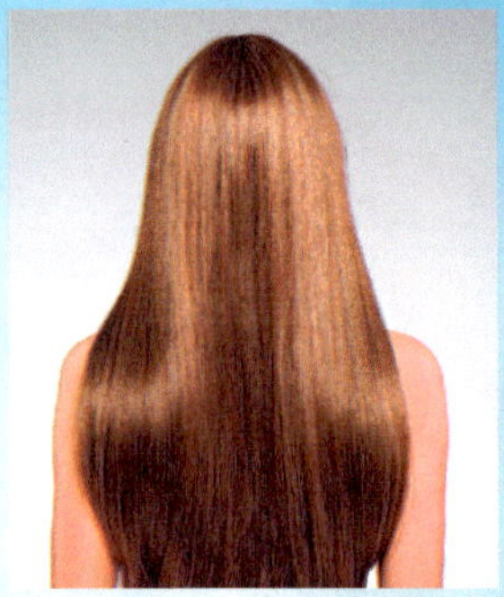

No More Bad Habits

First, understand that correcting your bad eating habits and doing a detox, which I will speak about a little further in the book, will get you started on your path to optimal health.

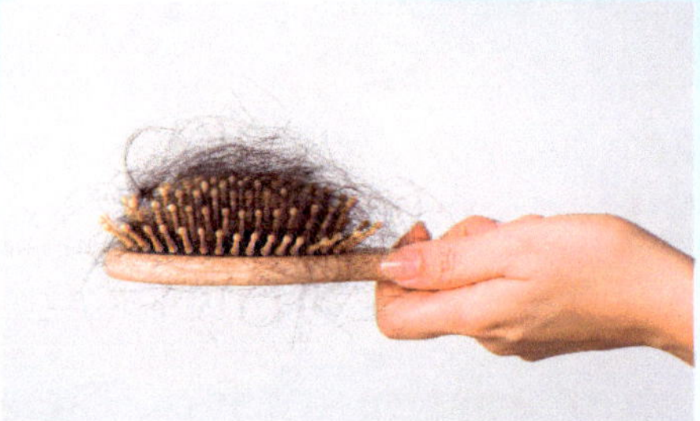

Crazy Hair

I usually have a problem with dryness and now dealing with crazy grey hair as we all know how frustrating it can be that many women go with shorter styles to be able to handle better.

Brushing your hair before bed helps with growth and stress because it stimulates the scalp. Three-month trims also stimulate growth. As a child, I always wanted to grow my hair, and I never wanted to cut it, but my hair grew so slowly.

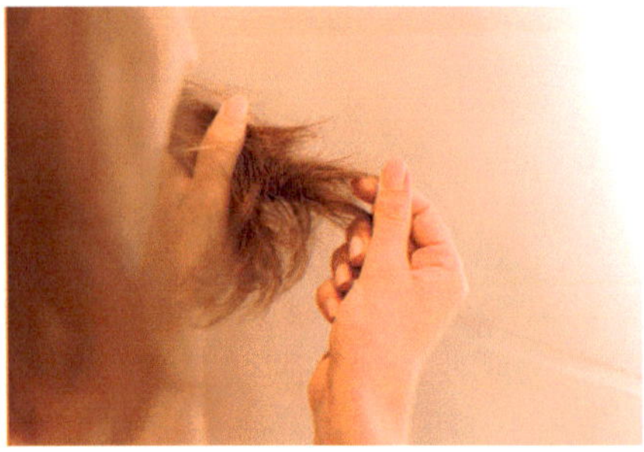

Amazing Tricks

Well, here are some amazing tricks to help strengthen, soften, and alleviate dryness:

My favorite hair mask, believe me, is Mayonnaise.

For hair growth, almond oil, rosemary, frankincense, and cloves work well.

Look for instructions at the end of the book, where I will add this and a few key recipes you will love. Rice water is absolutely the best hair rinse that leaves your hair soft.

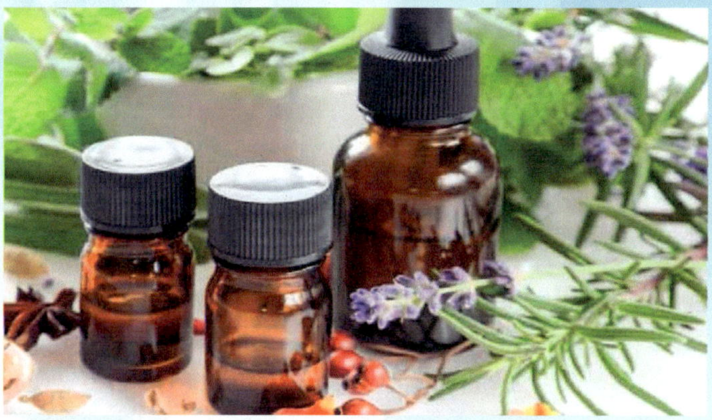

Rice Water Method

Hair should be washed with warm water, preferably spring water if possible, and always rinse off last with icy water. This matters because warm water opens the hair shaft just as it opens the pores on your skin.

Icy water closes the shaft to protect the hair from breakage like a protective seal. When possible, use cold rice water to rinse. Rice water will last three days in the fridge in a glass jar and is easily made by saving the water after cooking your rice; the type of rice does not matter.

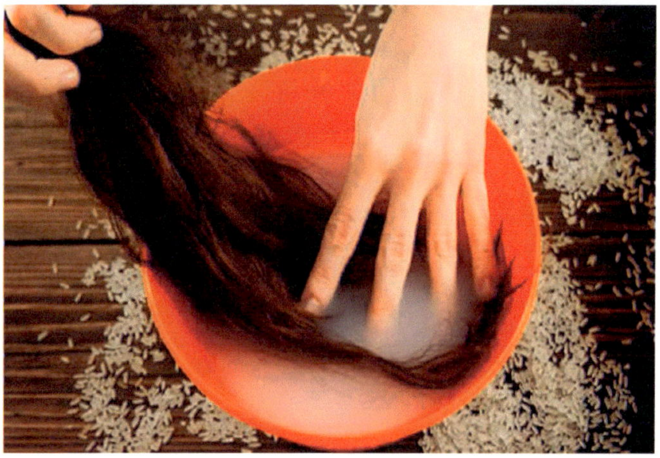

The Growth

Going forward, I cannot wait to trim it because it grows like weeds now that I have been working on all these changes that I am sharing with you from my own experience and those I have helped by sharing this information. Grow your hair and nails by eating low fat Jell-O.

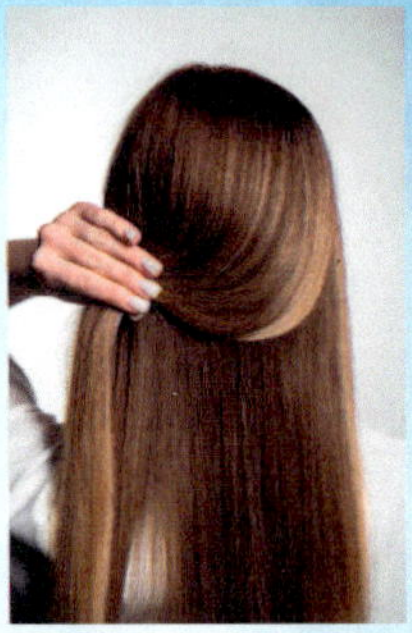

Eyelash Care

Grow your eyelashes back or longer with castor oil and a new toothbrush. It takes a little time and dedication on your part, but you are worth the effort, and I have also even seen eyebrows grow back with patients.

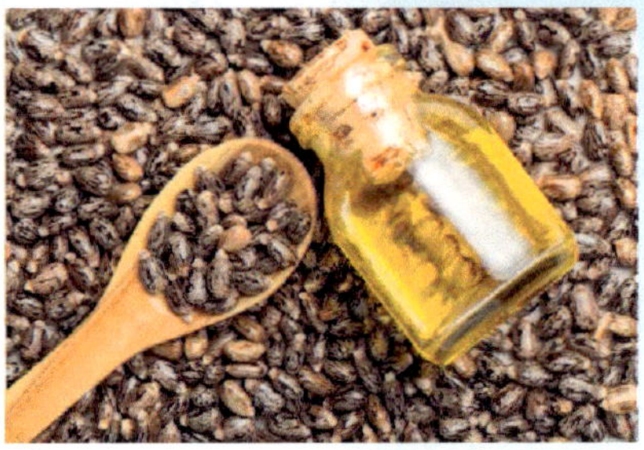

Lip Care

Now, for your lips, do not be afraid to brush them when cleaning your teeth. It stimulates the blood flow and softens off dead skin. Dry lips are a sign of dehydration, and I will give my recommendation as to which source of hydration I prefer and how to enhance your water intake.

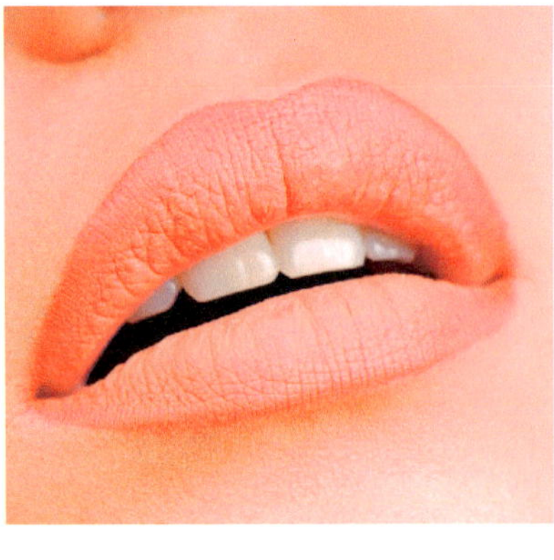

Healthy Ears

Let us not forget our ears and be careful when using ear cleaners as sometimes they can have the opposite effect and pack the wax in instead of removing it, which in time will cause a build up and hearing loss. Once, I had to go to the doctor to remove the cotton piece at the end of the ear cleaner that got stuck in my ear drum. It was no fun.

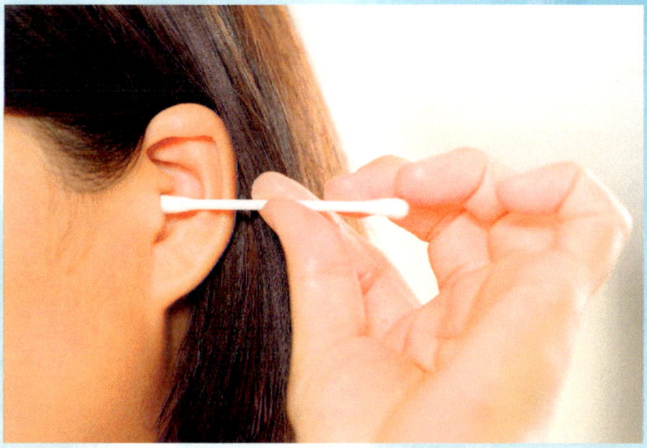

Treating Earache

This week, as I draft this book, I have an ear infection from a lovely cold my children shared with me, and earache is something else, let me tell you.

I took one regular cooking onion with its skin on and put it to boil in a pot for ten minutes. Then I removed it carefully and cooled it for a few minutes because you want it to be hot still. I cut it in half and wrapped each half in a cotton washcloth, but you could also use double paper towels so it's not directly touching the skin.

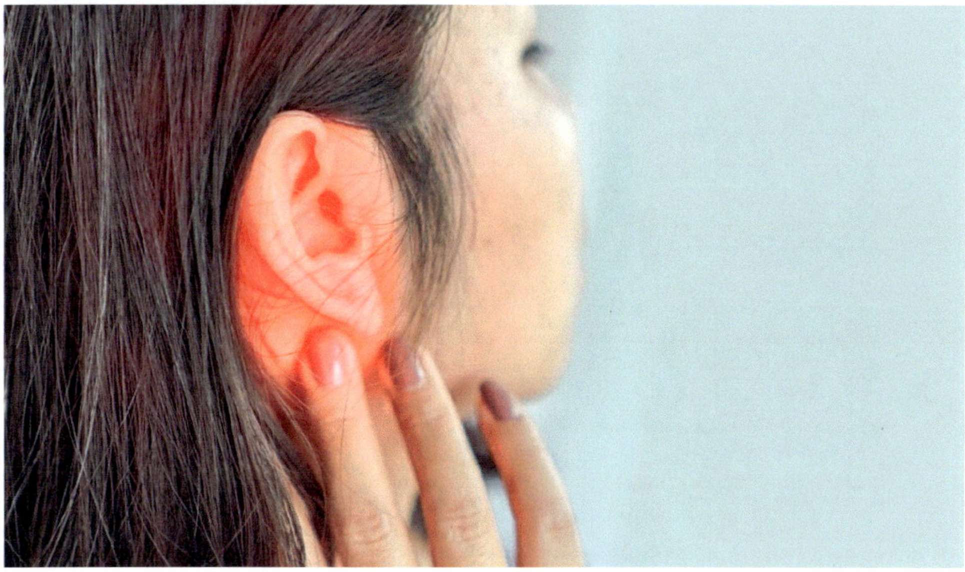

Treatment Continues

I took a normal towel and wrapped it around my head and made a fold around the front part before wrapping to create a pocket like wrap to place the open sides of the onions wrapped towards the ear in each pocket over my ears. This is wonderful for ear pain, especially for kids who cannot sleep from the pain.

I did these two nights in a row, leaving on for about an hour. It held the heat and drew out the pain – the whole hour was wonderful.

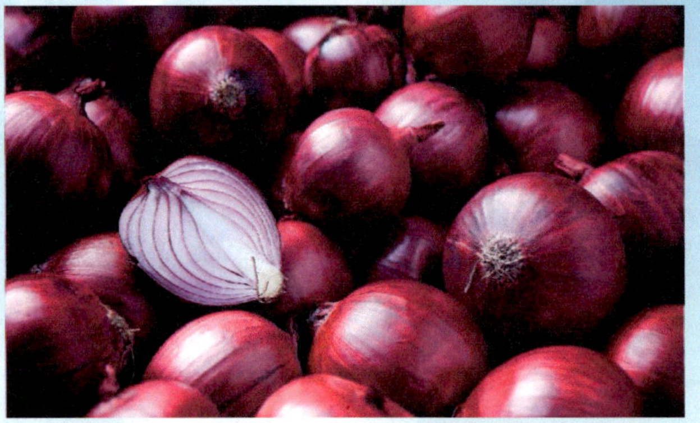

Treating Shaving Rash

How about shaving? Rash is not that fun. Well, guess what? It's baby aspirin, non-coated original. Place two or three in your hand, add a drop of water to make a paste, and rub over. After shaving, leave for a few minutes. Then rinse. No more bumps, ingrown hairs, rash, nothing perfect, right?

Inflammatory and heals the skin. Wait until I tell you why I prefer Aspirin when I mostly avoid using medicine, choosing natural first.

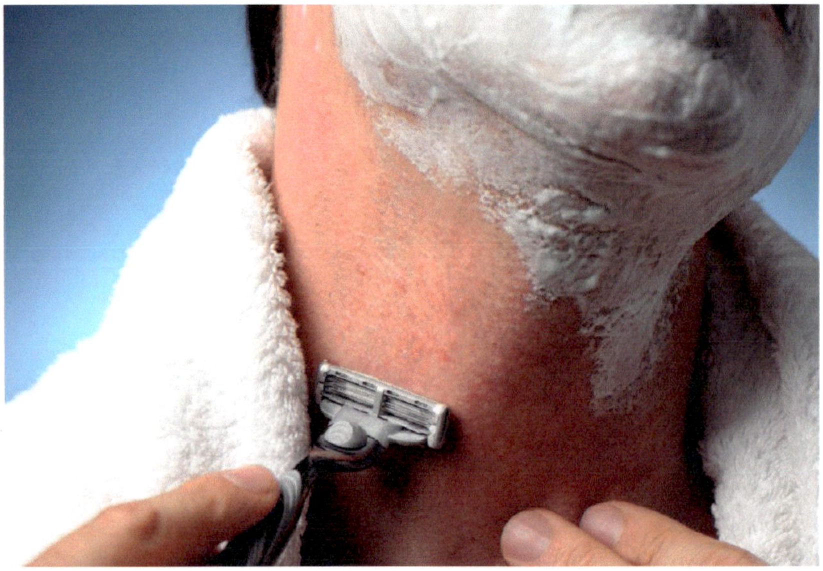

Tips & Tricks

Nail Care

Yellowing nails try soaking in old school brown mouthwash not only will it help kill bacteria on hands and feet it helps remove the yellowing.

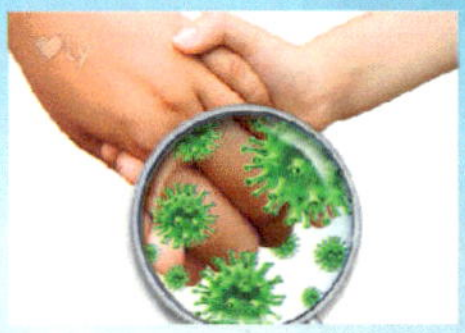

Healthy Breathing

Smokers or chest congestion Mullein tea crazy stuff, this will clear out your lungs like nothing I have seen before. Add honey for benefits.

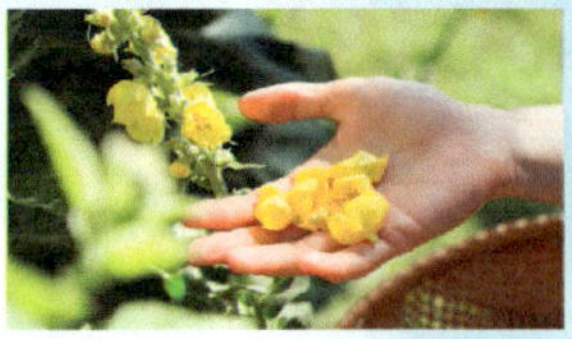

Razor Burns

2 baby aspirin with drop of water to make a paste add topical.

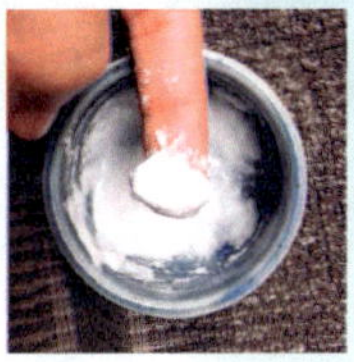

Teeth Whitening

Whiten teeth once a month to ensure you don't remove any enamel. Drop Peroxide with a sprinkle of salt and baking soda and brush softly over stains on teeth try to avoid the gums as salt can make the gums sensitive.

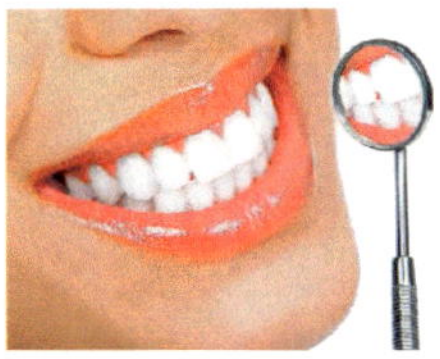

No More Warts

Get rid of warts by using hand sanitizer and a band aid make sure to change daily.

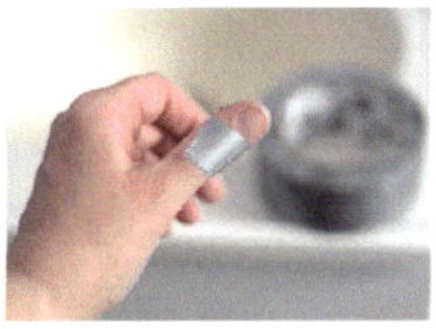

More Skin Tips

Soften your skin: Add sea salts like Himalayan, Celtic or Grey salt to your baths.

Acne prone skin: Get rid of pimples by using the pear soap I suggested along with peppermint tea which also helps menstrual cramps.

To Lose weight: One shot glass of half freshly squeezed lemon, half teaspoon of cayenne and olive oil or coconut your choice daily first thing in morning after one glass of water.

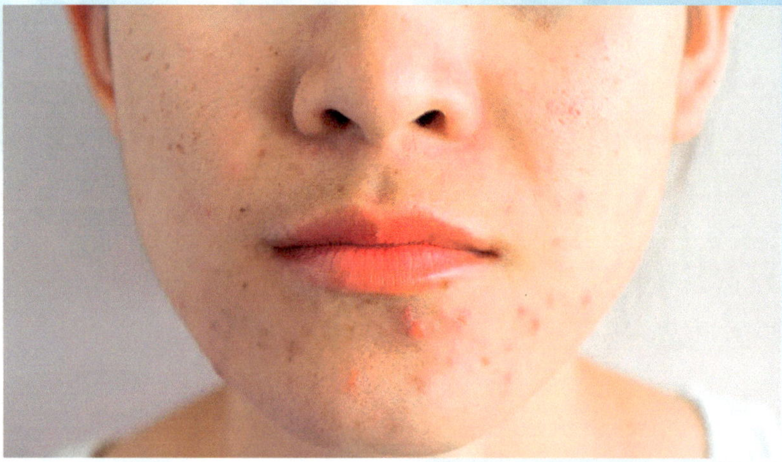

Oil Tips

Coconut and olive oil for hair smoothing just a drop in your hands apply well dry so you can control amount applied.

Castor oil not only will moisturize your entire body, but it will help eyelashes grow back with a new soft toothbrush go over daily softly gentle with eyes.

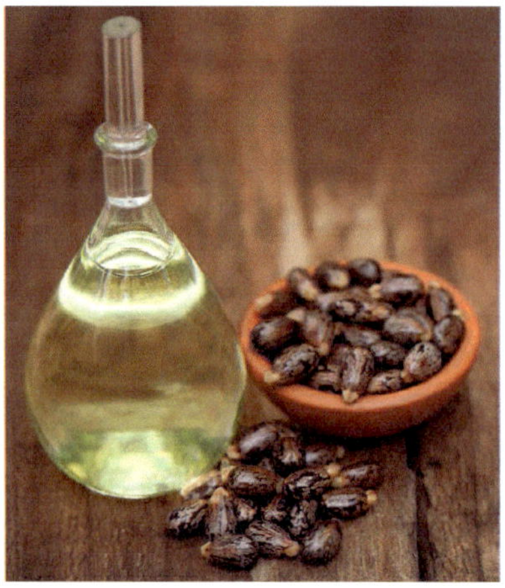

Save From Stroke

Save a life if someone is having a stroke you can put cayenne on their tongue, and this will help until help arrives. If coherent follow with glass of water. No, they will not feel the heat from cayenne during stroke.

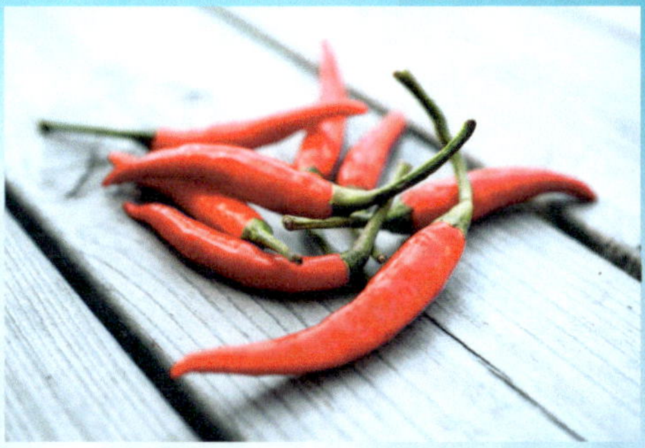

Hair Growth

Grow hair with almond oil cloves rosemary basil using half cup of oil, teaspoon of cloves and two teaspoons of rosemary and place in glass jar for 24 hours then use after washing concentrating on scalp. I do suggest a detox always first as blockages could be the main cause for hair thinning and loss.

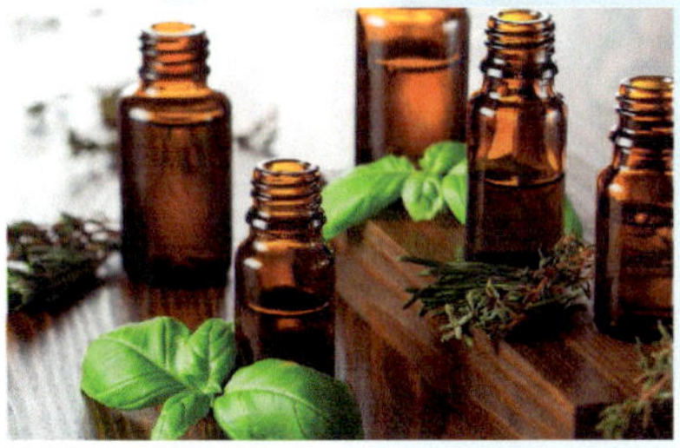

Cancer Cure

Help cure cancer with soursop tea and apricot seeds organic of course. Take two daily and only two apricot seeds daily for 15 days then break two to three weeks before trying again. Do your research this one is outstanding!

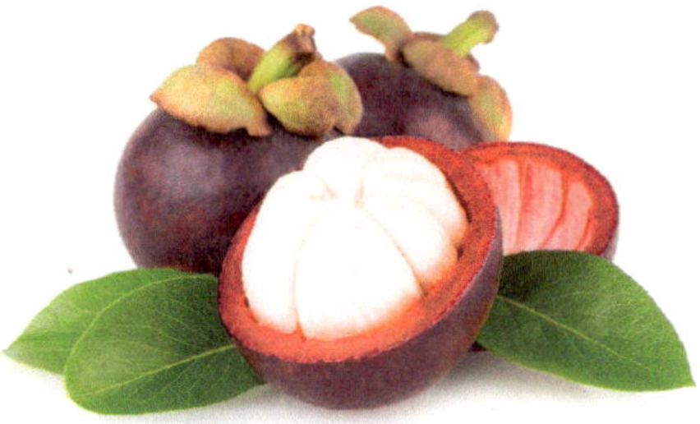

RECIPES

Cold and Flu Syrup

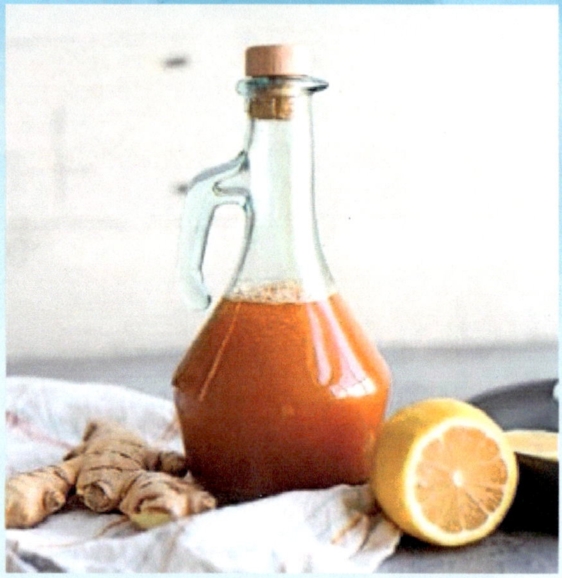

Elderberry cold syrup one bag of frozen or fresh elderberries approx. four cups add 10 cups of water handful of cloves and 5 sticks of cinnamon and boil then turn off and add 500ml of organic honey stir in well and the fill your glass jars cool and refrigerate for three months and have family members take two teaspoons daily during the cold and flu season.

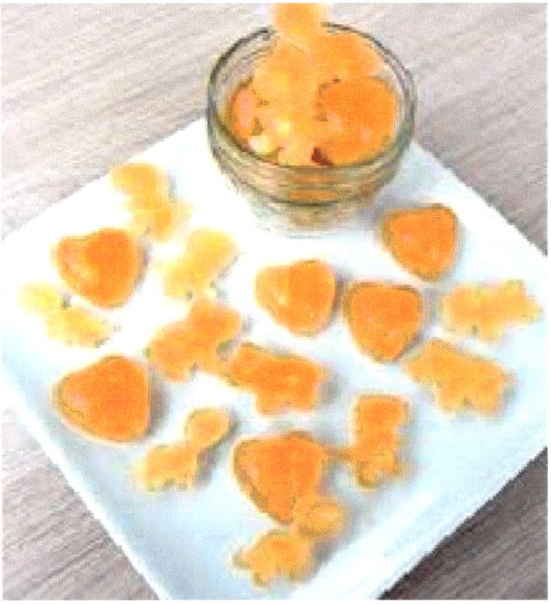

Cold and Flu Gummies

Bonus: turn your Elderberry cold syrup into gummies easily by adding gelatin, follow package instructions, and pour in teddy shaped trays and cool in fridge. Pop out, then place in glass jars. Both the syrup and gummies must be kept in fridge and last for three months. P.S they never last that long my kids love them and effortless way to get vitamins daily safely.

Homemade Toothpaste

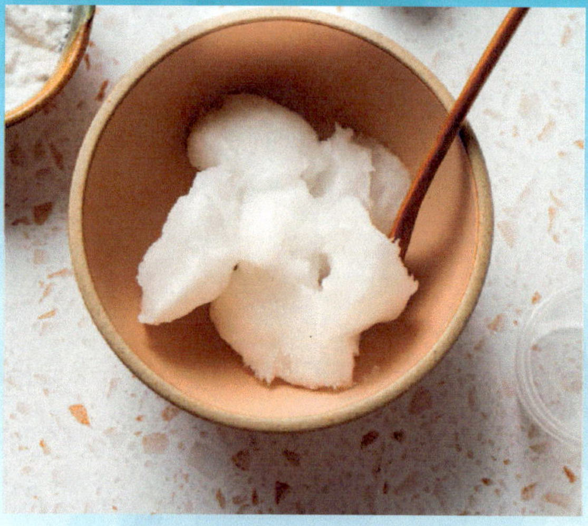

¾ tsp glycern,1 teaspoon shea butter, ¼ tsp castor oil, ¼ beeswax, ¼ coconut oil, ½ tsp bentonite clay, 1 tsp activated charcoal, two drops of mint oil or rosemary depending on flavor choice is yours. Mix all ingredients in a bowl the fill small glass jar for convenient.

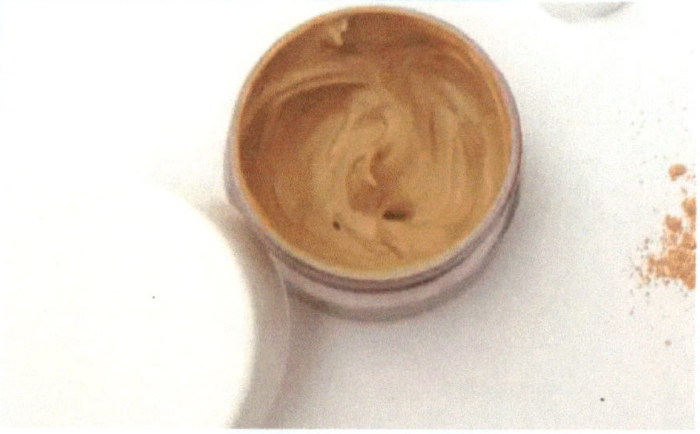

Liquid Foundation

2 tsp zinc oxide 1/8 gold mica dust, 1 tsp rhassoul powder (you can select a clay that matches your skin tones, 2tsp fine ground coco (adjust to optimize your color).

Candles

Candles are bee's wax and a wick and that is it. These wax candles are better for your health to burn.

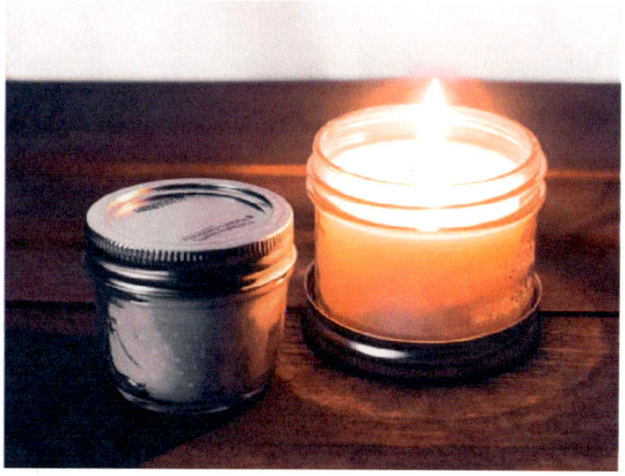

Blueberry Smoothie

1 cup blueberries

1 carrot peeled and chopped.

1 teaspoon wheatgerm or flex seeds

1 cup of almond milk (or any desired milk)

1tbs honey or maple syrup (optional for sweetness) Ice cubes (option al for chilled smoothie) Instructions:

1 Place all ingredients in blender
2 Blend until smooth creamy
3 Taste and adjust sweetness if desired, by adding honey or maple.
4 To boost it I add a bit more ice and a sprinkle of cinnamon.

Before trying any detox, you must understand that you need to have a binder kale or greens with every meal. |Detox and fasting well pregnant is not recommended. You should always speak to your doctor. When doing a detox, it has been recommended for at least 10 days with 5 days off.

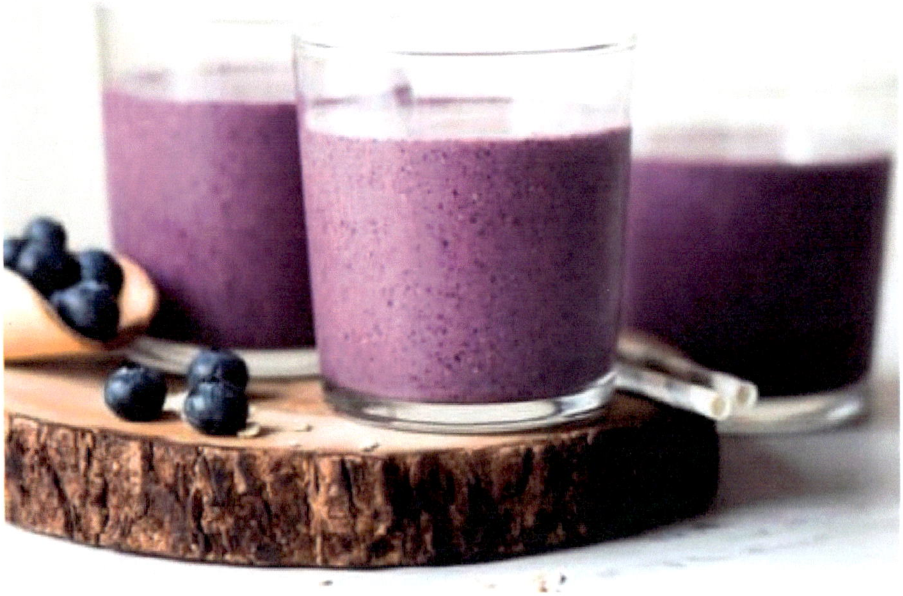

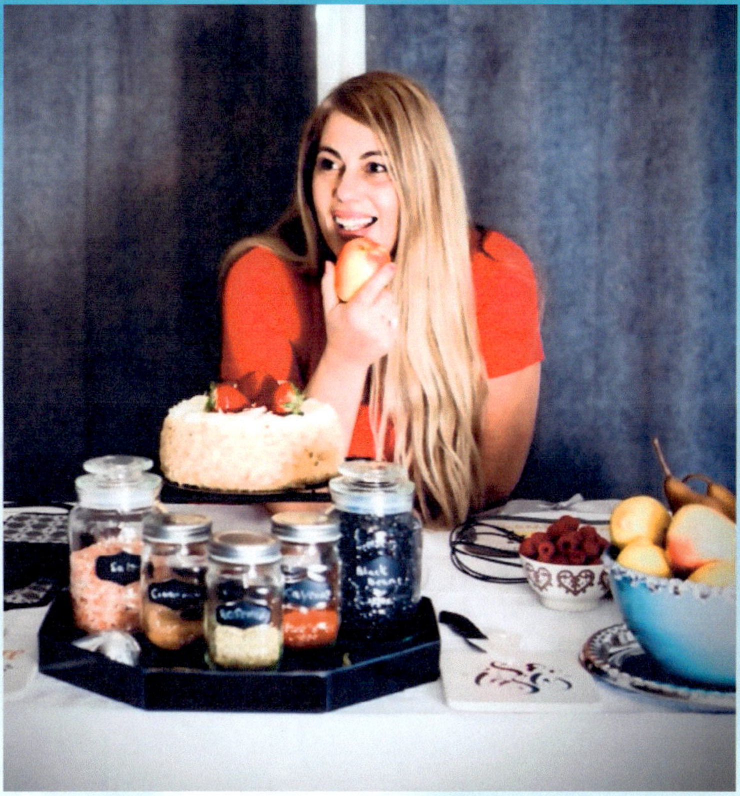

Talk about Diets

Have you ever known someone who was on a diet, and they lost weight but now they look older? I think many people would say yes and that is because they restricted themselves of vitamins and minerals, they need to be healthy skin hair nails. When your calorie restricts your taking away necessary nutrients your skin, hair, nails need. So important to do properly with your doctor's advice.

Detox methods

Lemon drops

1 whole lemon, ½ cucumber, few sprigs of mint, tsp of honey add ice to a blender.

Dragon's den

1 tablespoon of organic lemon, 2 tablespoons of maple syrup, ½ tea spoon cayenne

Cucumber water for weight loss

One cucumber, one whole lemon, 8 sprigs of mint to two-liter jug of spring water or alkaline water

Detox lemonade

Juice of one lemon, tsp honey pinch of cayenne, pinch of ginger, pinch of ground cloves, one cup of boil water drink as a tea

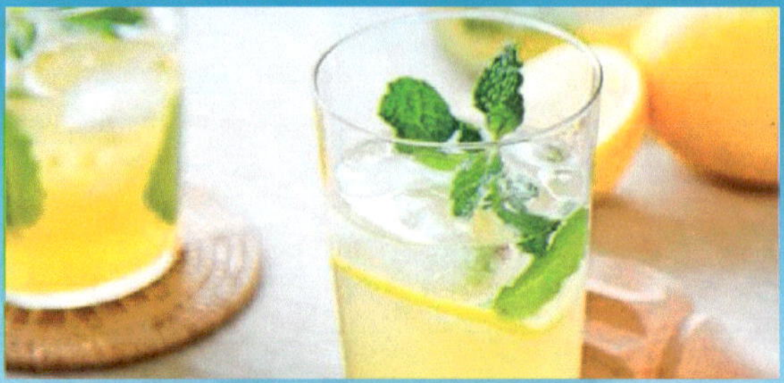

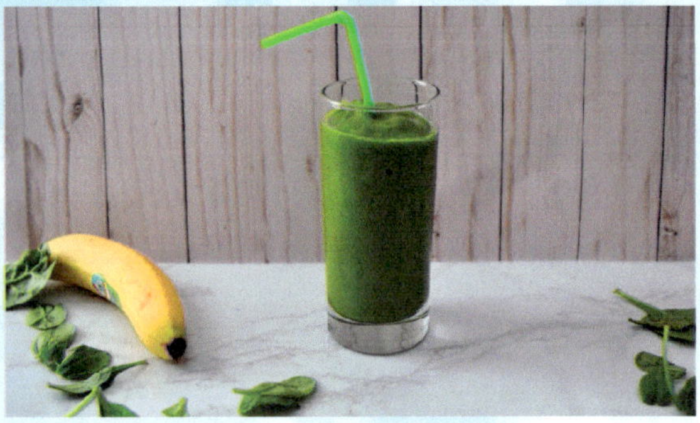

Island detox

Raspberries one cup, one lemon, handful of mint, one tsp honey, piece of lavender or tsp rosewater Add to one liter of spring water or filtered water of your choice.

More detox

Activated charcoal, zeolite, bentonite clay, chlorella, parsley.

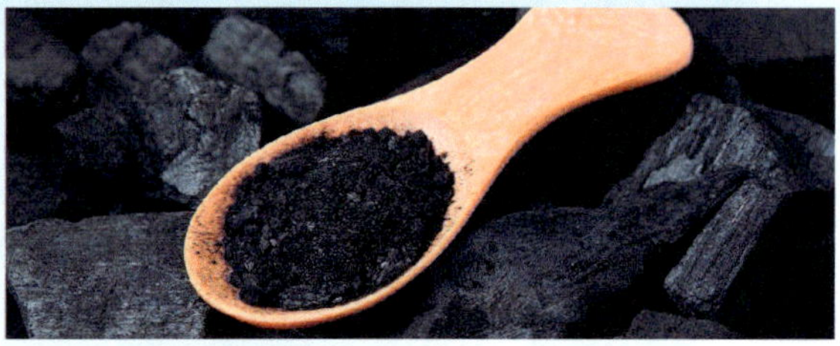

Something about water

The best waters for our body in my opinion are spring water or alkaline water which I believe is optimal as it balances our stomach PH level at 9.5 which is good for digestion, but always ask your doctor as people with acid reflux would do better on spring water or filtered.

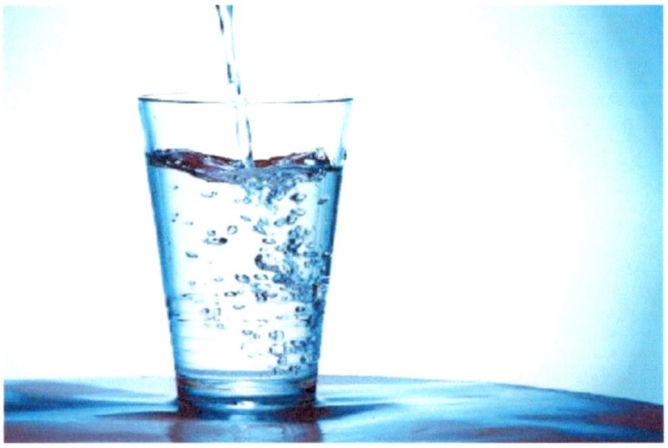

Oils

Coconut oil best for cooking, frying, hair, skin, laxative, healing cuts, sunscreen, oil pulling. But it may not be suitable for people with allergies.

Almond oil best for skin, hair growth, bath, tanning lotion but not for people with nut allergies. Avocado oil helps nutrient absorption, healthy fat, omega-6, omega –3, reduces cholesterol Olive oil best for cooking, hair, skin, makeup remover, soften meats, dressing, jarring.

Butter is delicious best for baking, topping, lite frying.

Blood cleaning ability, 3 sticks of celery and one lime juiced twice a week drink cold.

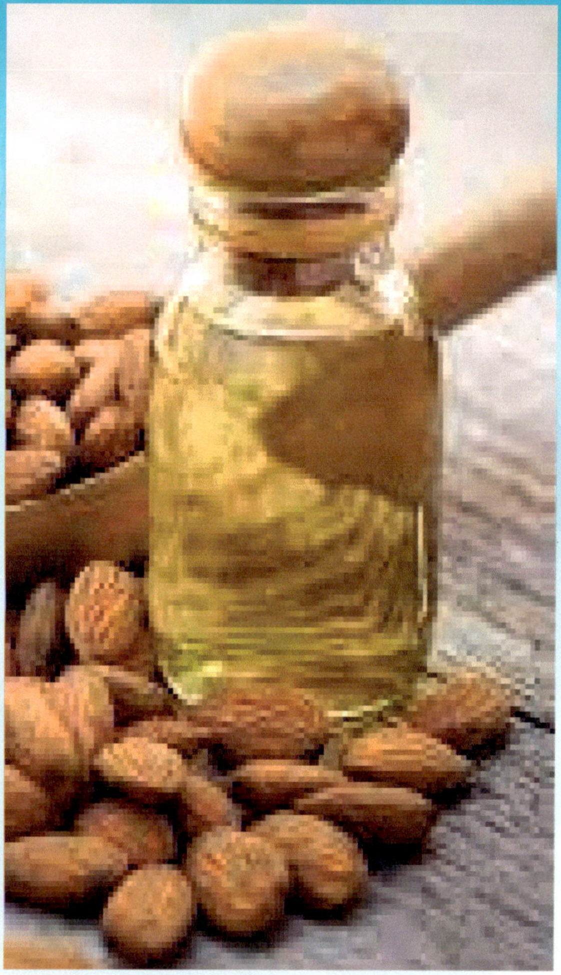

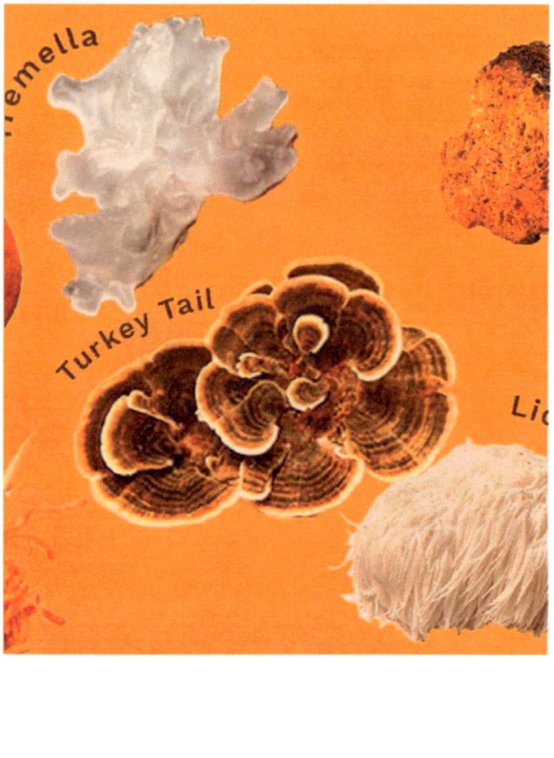

Interesting Mushrooms

Did you know that turkey tail mushrooms are an approved treatment for cancer in Japan! Might be a wonderful mushroom to add to our well living eating.

Chaga mushrooms also assist with cancer.

Loins main is an incredible mushroom for memory retention and let me just tell you how amazing this stuff is gold and works like a gem.

Apricot Seeds

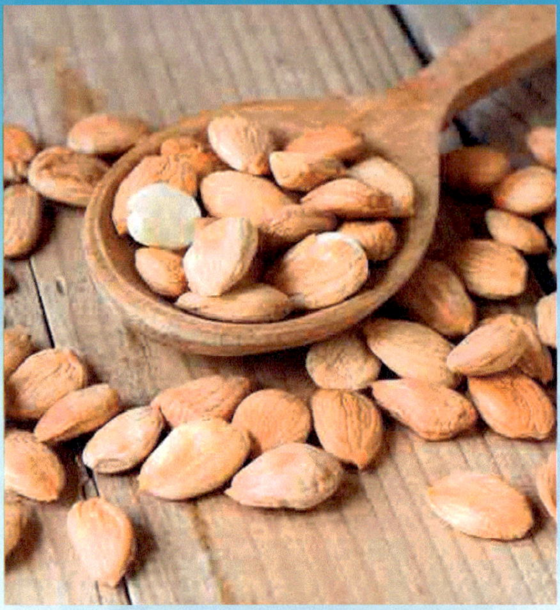

I have heard many interesting stories of people with cancer using all the above-mentioned along with apricot seeds and soursop to cure their own cancer several times in a natural way always worth trying.

Sea moss and kelp will help my ladies with fertility.

Kelp: Helps with keeping use youthful and good for fertility.

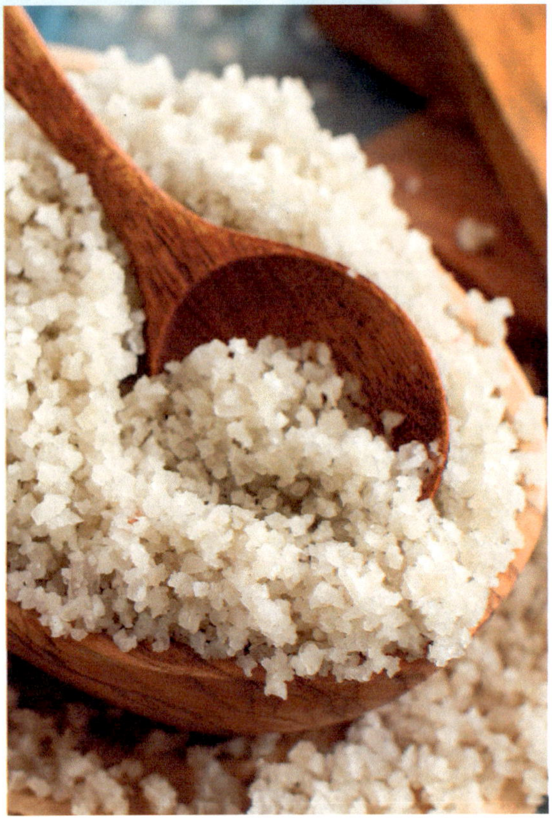

Salts

Celtic salt sometimes referred to as grey salt as well and Himalayan salt are great for your health and give you most of your trace minerals by using them daily, one granular of salt on the tongue before drinking water can help your cells absorb water into cells and help with hydration. I do recommend using these salts.

I also recommend using filtered water spring water and alkaline water as many tap waters contain fluoride and chemicals. It makes a difference on your hair and skin too.

Kala Walla Root

Kala Walla root cures 30 chronic diseases and protects the skin from cancer.

Hair Growth

Batana oil, people claim hair growth within nine days saying that it reverses alopecia and balding in days. Rosemary.

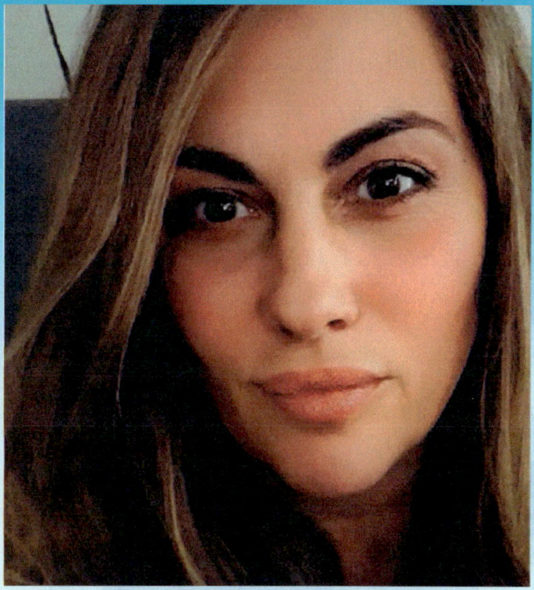

Top 10 parasite destroyers

Pumpkin seeds, oregano oil, clove oil, black walnut, grapefruit seeds extract, olive leaf extract, wormwood, garlic and onions, papaya seeds, apricot seeds

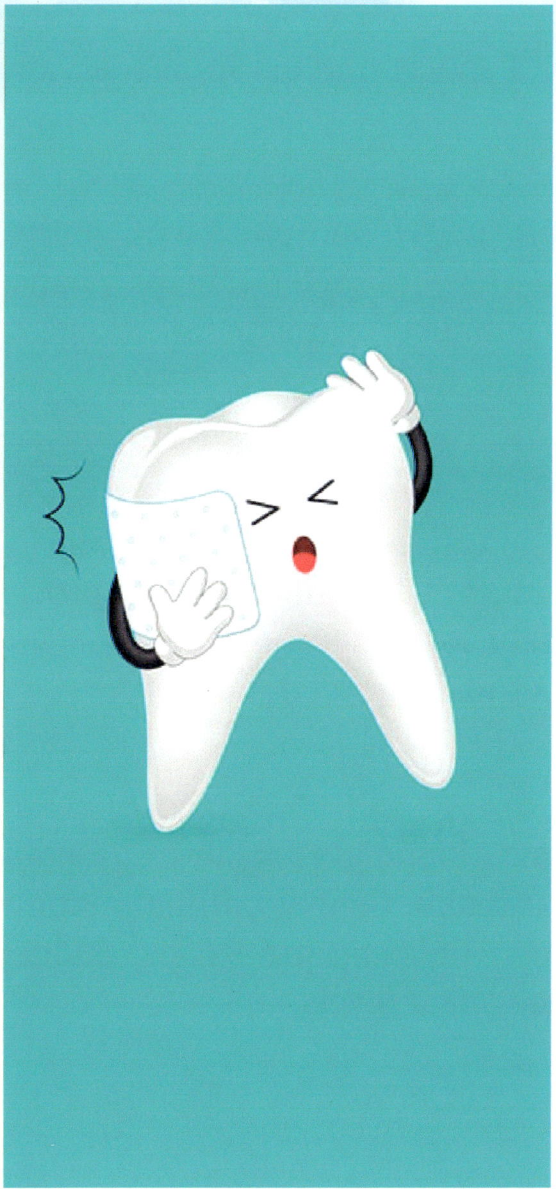

Tooth Aches

grab a handful of cloves and put them in spring water, I usually put about a half cup of them in my water bottle let sit few hours to soak. This clove water can be saved and used for up to a month room temperature. Simply rinse hold in your mouth long as you can swishing around the mouth then spit out do not swallow. I have used many times works amazing fast and lasted. Clove oils and water were used back to relieve pain during dental work ask your dentist.

My dentist said that they do not like telling people about this because it worked so well that some people do not get the dental work necessary for them because they no longer feel any pain. You should always get necessary work done and not avoid.

Food with Benefits and Superfoods

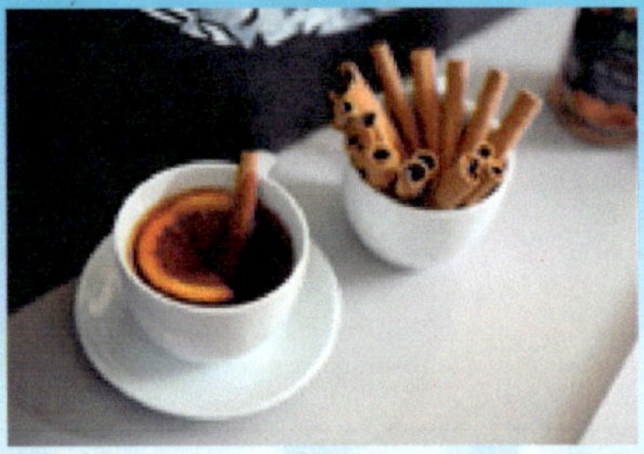

Cinnamon Anti-fungal, antioxidant, anti-inflammatory, anti-bacteria, Anti-viral, improves insulin sensitivity, medicinal properties, protect against heart disease, lower blood sugars, beneficial effects on neurodegenerative diseases, reducing cancer growth, Ceylon true cinnamon, small doses work best.

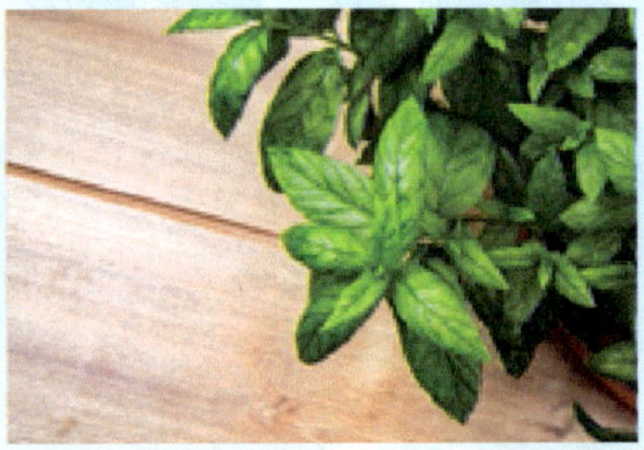

Peppermint cramps, acne, flavoring toothpaste or drinks, irritable bowel syndrome, sinus infections, headaches, digestive peppermint water for constipation. Peppermint oil for aches and pains, nausea.

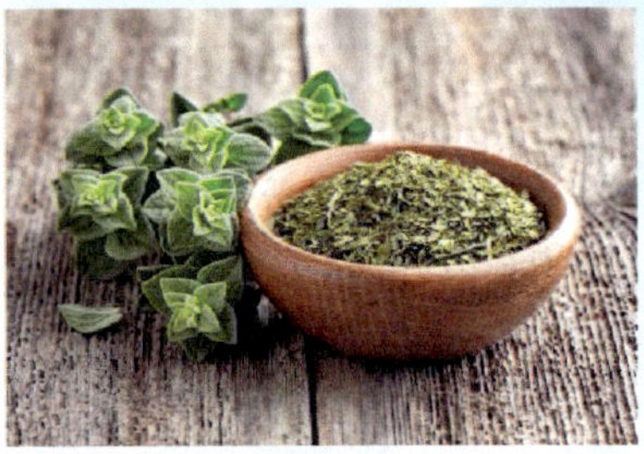

Oregano anti-fungal, antimicrobial, antiviral, reduce cough, prevents bacteria, helps balance hormones, mood enhancer, parasite infections.

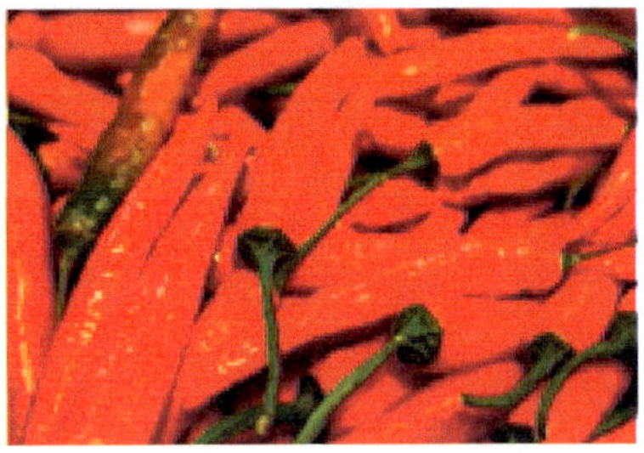

Cayenne nasal congestion, sinus pain, headache, vitamin A, B, C, E, antioxidant, improves heart health, weight loss, digestion, blood sugar, immunity, circulation flow erection.

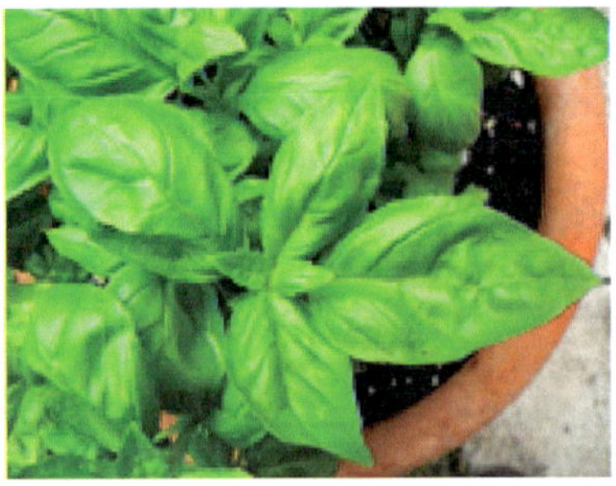

Basil maintains blood glucose levels, mental health, boost health skin benefits, inflammation, depression, cancer fighting properties, kidney health, lower blood sugar levels.

Food with Benefits and Superfoods

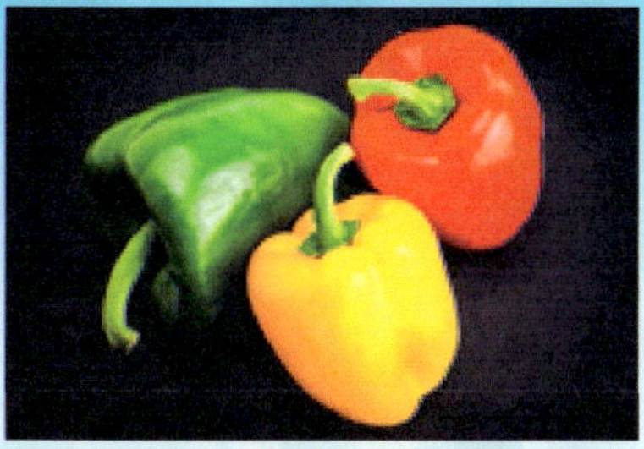

Peppers low calorie, vitamins A, C, folic acid, fiber, lowers blood sugars, memory loss, delay aging, less hungry during the day.

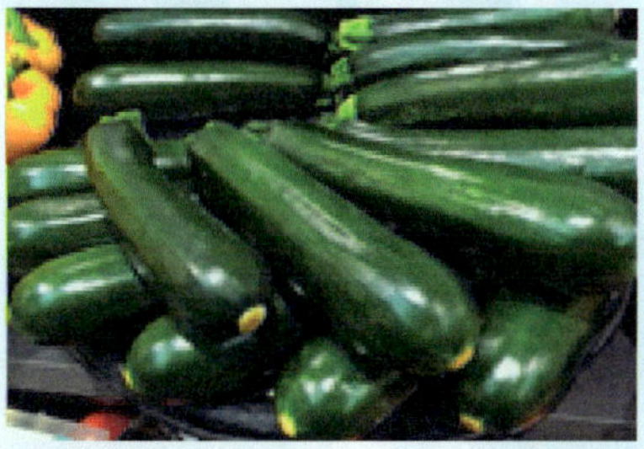

Zucchini Immune system, eye health, lowers cholesterol, strong bone health, gut microbiomes, blood pressure.

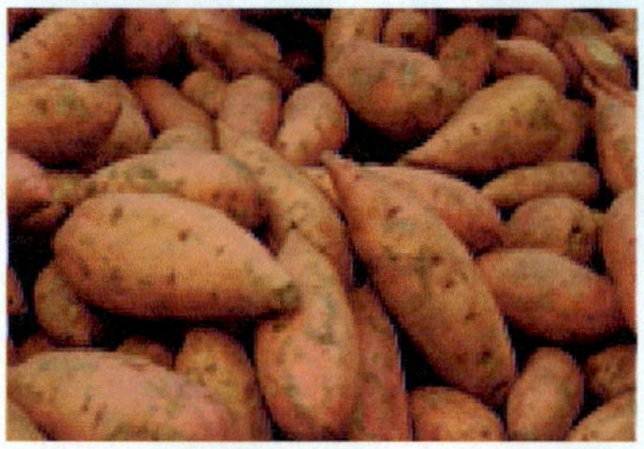

Sweet potato support weight loss, protects against chronic diseases, lowers blood sugars, protein, fiber, protects free radical damage, vitamins A, B, C and trace minerals.

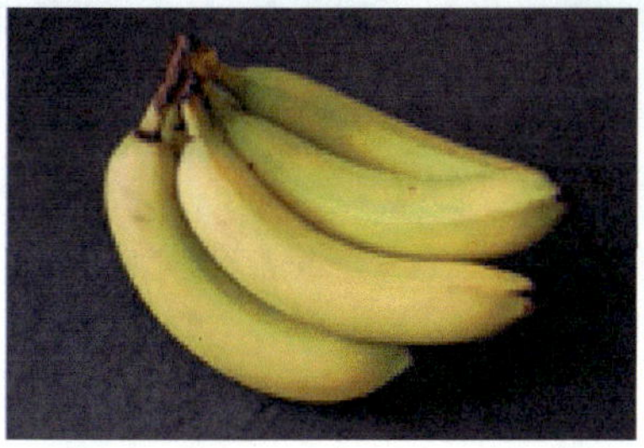

Banana aids in digestion, fiber, heart health, blood pressure, gastrointestinal issues, energy, skin, vitamin C, low calories, antioxidants.
Best eaten before lunch keeps you full.

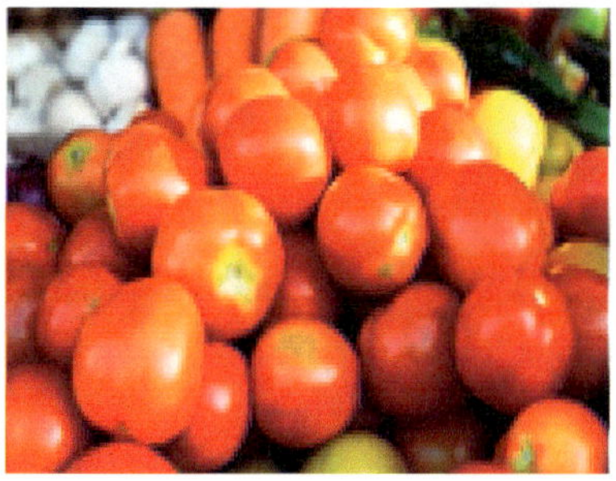

Tomato brain health, heart health, gut, vitamin C, potassium, lycopene,
Antioxidant, lowers cholesterol, brightens skin, cancer fighting.

Food with Benefits and Superfoods

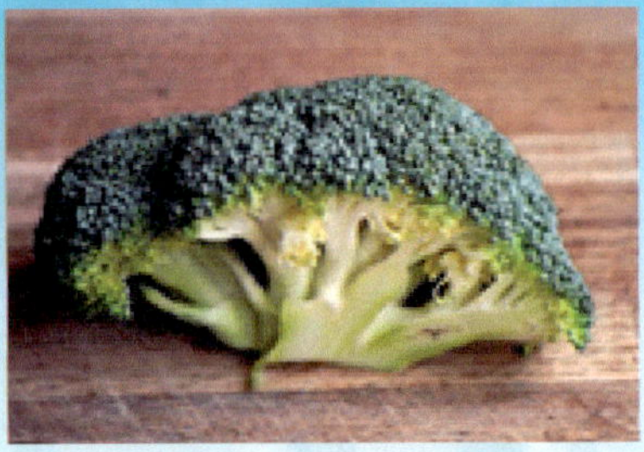

Broccoli bone health, inflammation, protects against cancer, Controls blood sugars, aid digestion, brain function, improves heart health, Fiber, iron, potassium, vitamin C, K, known to help the body absorb iron.

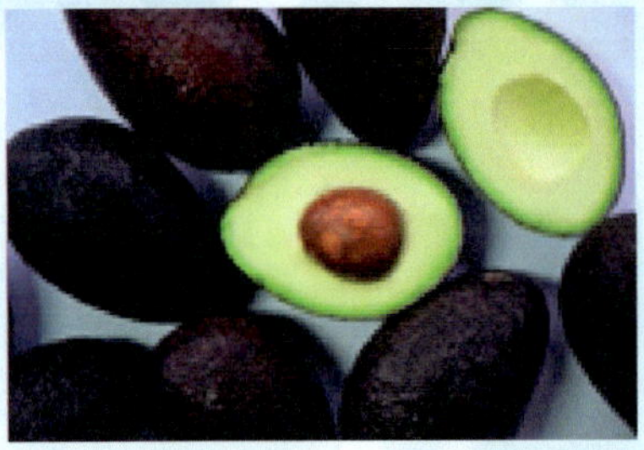

Avocado helps vision, moisturizing, preventing osteoporosis, fetal health.
Digestion, depression, detoxification, fiber, immune system, anti-microbial
Healthy fat.

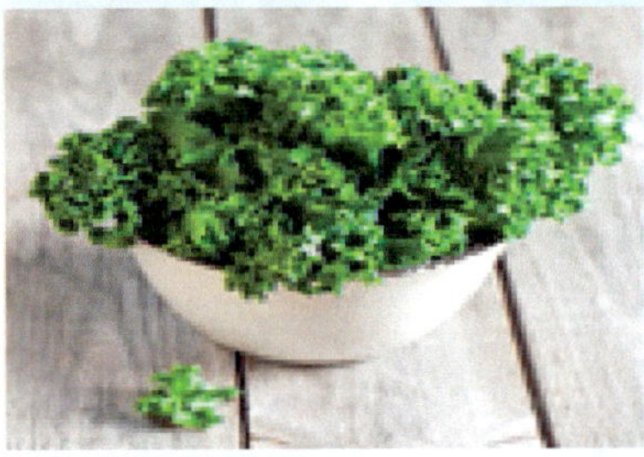

Kale reducing risks of various types of cancer, regulating blood pressure, vitamin A, K, C, folate, potassium, calcium, magnesium. Those who should avoid people with oxalate-containing kidney stones or take blood thinners.

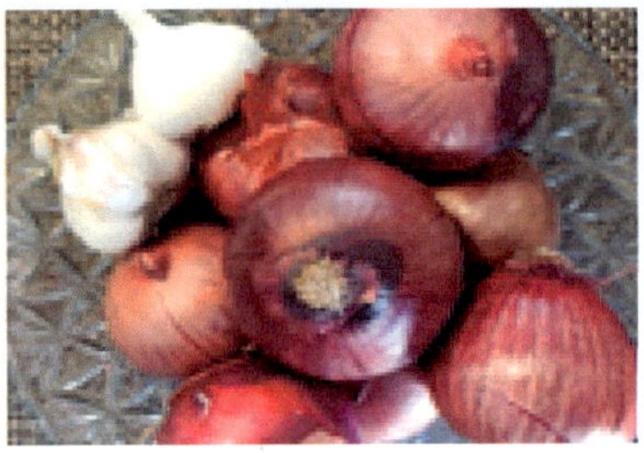

Onion's collagen production, protects cells, immune cells, iron absorption, potassium, vitamins C, B6, cellular functions, fluid balance, muscle contraction, kidney function, reduce heart disease, 17 types of flavonoids, blood sugar levels, bone density.

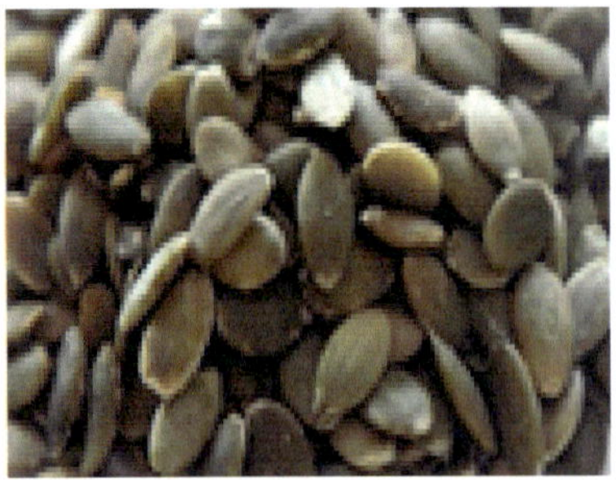

Pumpkin seeds help kill parasites, support prostate health, balance blood sugars, help fight cancer cell support called cell proliferation, heart health, promotes healthy cholesterol, menopause benefits hot flashes joint discomfort.

Food with Benefits and Superfoods

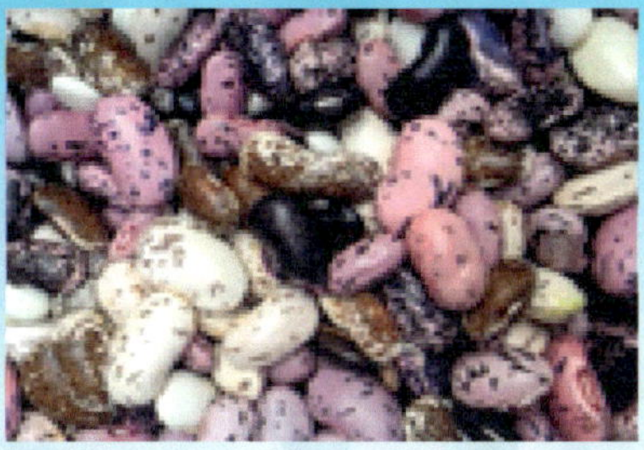

Beans great source of fiber, vitamins B, iron, copper, magnesium, manganese, zinc, phosphorus, low fat, folate.

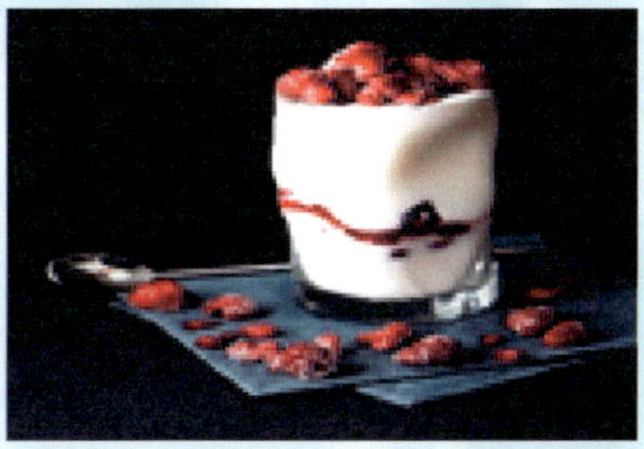

Yogurt high protein for muscle building, low sugar, calcium, live cultures, weight loss assistance, gastrointestinal infections, trace minerals.

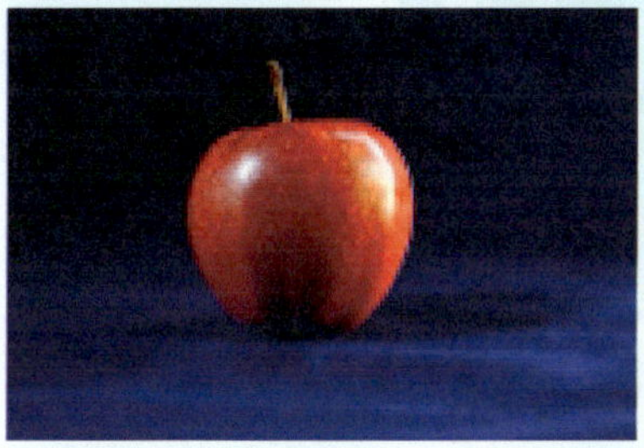

Apples Phytonutrient, cancer fighting properties and great source of Fiber. Stabilizes blood sugars, reduces blood pressure, eases inflammation, boost your microbiome, helps extend life, satisfies hunger, protects your heart, boost brain health, cancer fighting, lowers type two diabetes.

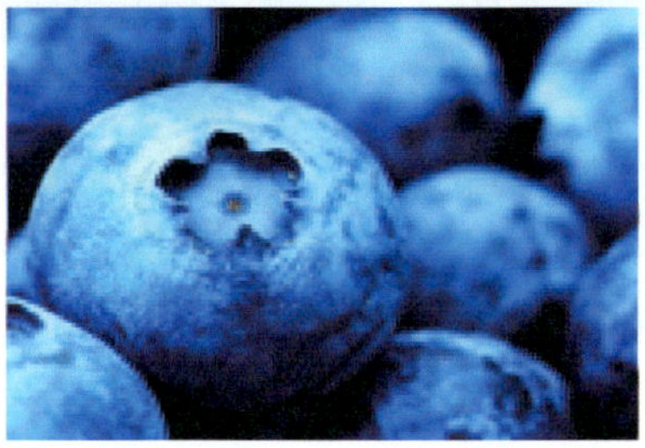

Blueberries cancer fighting properties, antioxidants super food, Brain health helps with recovery, vision, bone density, kidney health, digestion, cognition, heart health, lowers cholesterol, lowers blood pressure, controls blood sugars.

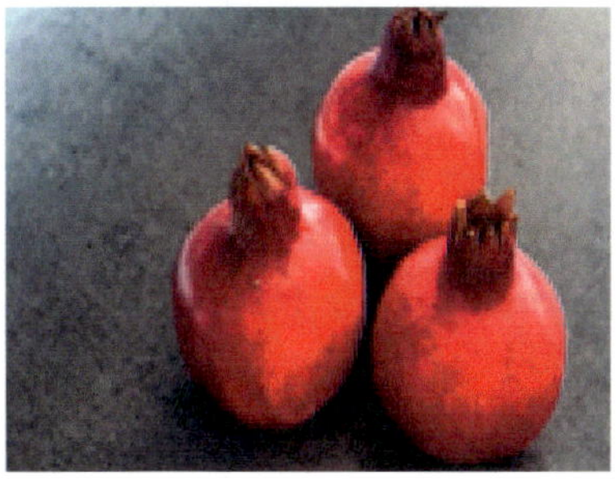

Pomegranate Vitamin C, D, A, E, cell regeneration, sun protection, anti aging properties, low calories snack, high fiber, potassium, boost immune system, helps joint tissues, bone loss, aids in digestion.

Food with Benefits and Superfoods

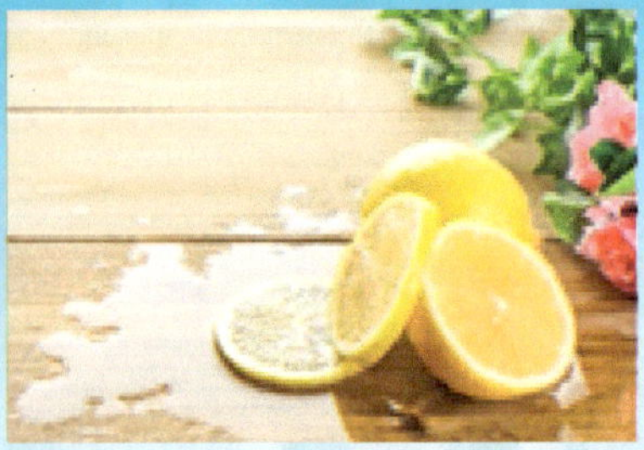

Lemon lightens hair and skin, remove dark underarm pits, weight control loss, reduced heart disease, digestive issues, (avoid with acid reflects) helps complexion, helps with iron absorption, packed with vitamin C, highly Alkalizing great in spring water.

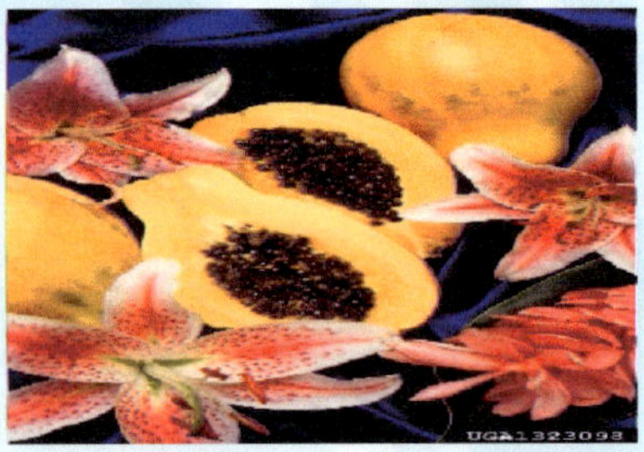

Papaya super food, parasite elimination, boosts immune system, helps protect heart disease, aids digestion, vitamin C, A, folate (B9) as well as trace amounts of B1, B3, E and K.

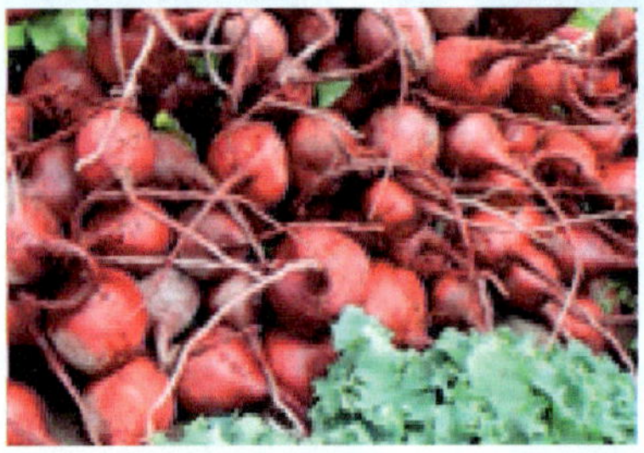

Red maca root powder is the best source, helps boost estrogen, energy, boost libido, sexual desires, mood improving, helps ladies with fertility.

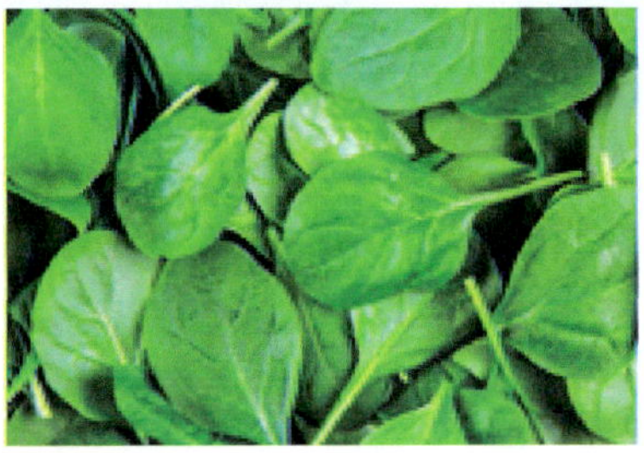

Spinach rich in iron, Vitamin E, C, potassium, magnesium, support immune function, digestive system, anti- cancer properties, inorganic nitrate, lower heart disease, helps arteries, eye health, reduces hypertension.

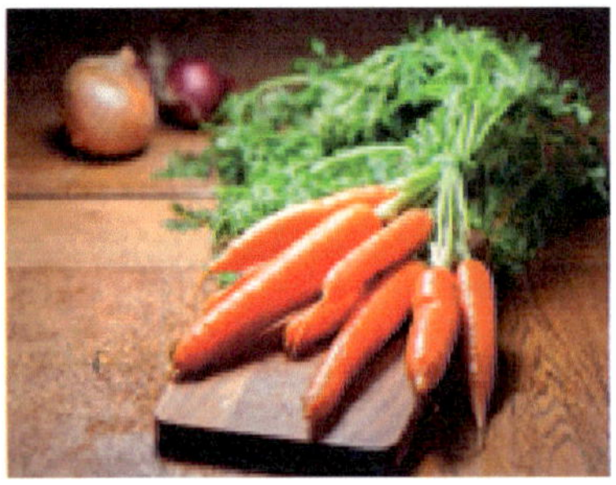

Carrot vision, balance blood sugars, weight management, lower cancer risks, helps regulate blood pressure, supports immunity, skin health, brain health, inflammation, Beta-carotene, potassium, antioxidants, and good source of vitamin A.

Food with Benefits and Superfoods

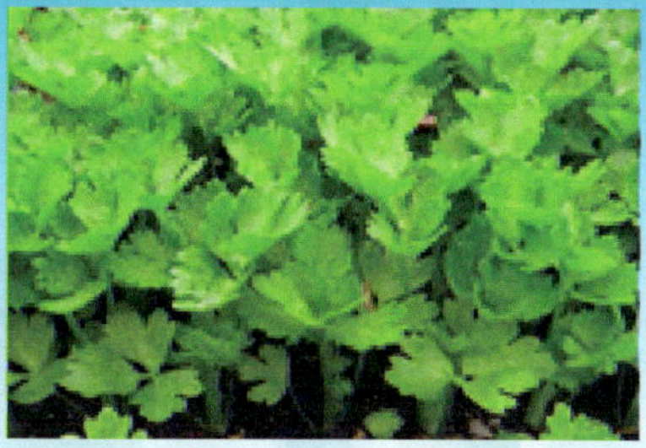

Celery has low calories, weight loss, high fiber, potassium, antioxidants, source of hydration 95% water, vitamin K, folate, boosts collagen production, protects against UV damage, skin detoxification, bowel movement. Helps clean the blood.

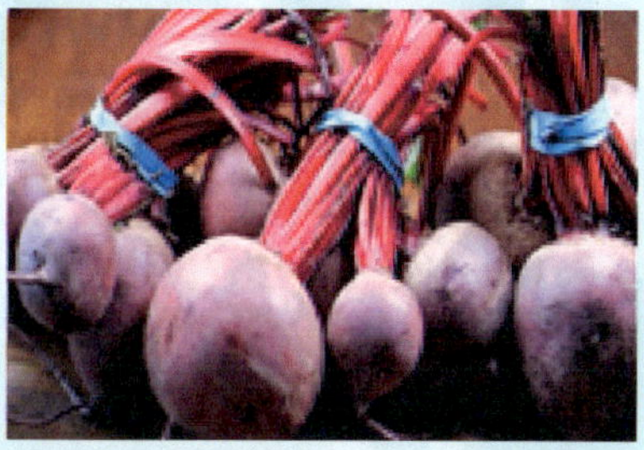

Beets brain health, heart health, digestive system, boosts athletic performance, antioxidants, B12, potassium, manganese, bone health, muscle health repair, high iron, B9, protein, copper, magnesium, vitamin C, B6, lowers blood pressure.

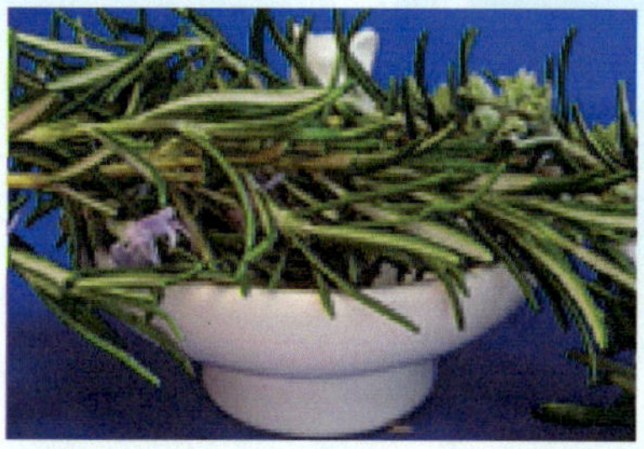

Rosemary blood circulation, immune system, antimicrobial, anti-inflammatory, anti-tumorigenic, anticipative, neuroprotective properties, neutralizing harmful free radicals, promotes hair growth, boosts production of red blood cells, mouth freshener, fights diseases and pathogens.

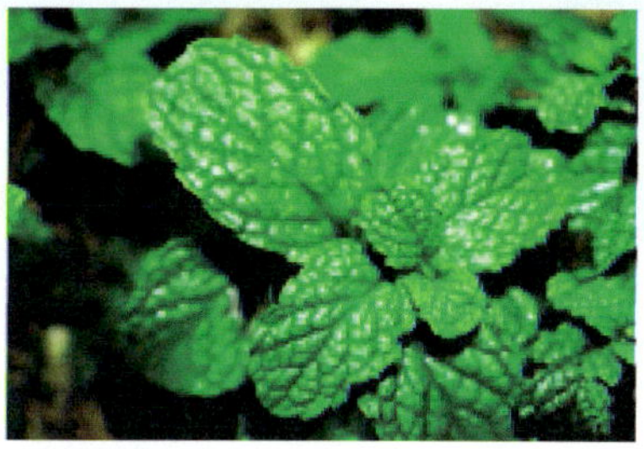

Mint brain health, stress relief, immune system, digestive health, mouth health and fresh, inflammatory properties, unclogs pores, vitamin A, eye health, indigestion, improves respiratory functions, helps stress depression, helps breast feeding pain, irritable bowel syndrome, improves weight loss, carotene prevents hair loss, helps ease allergy symptoms.

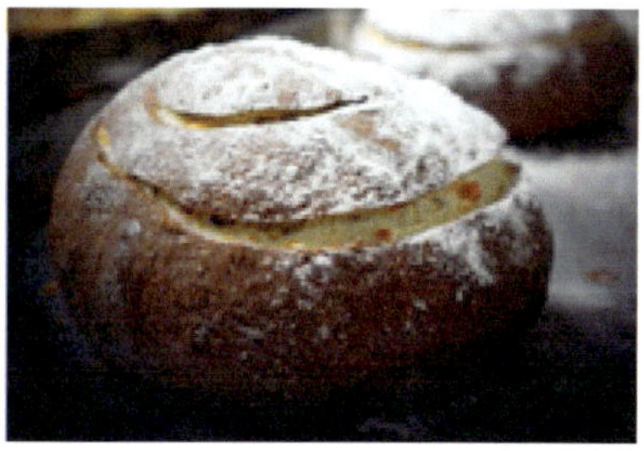

Breads recommended sour dough bread, Rye bread, Spelt bread.

Food with Benefits and Superfoods

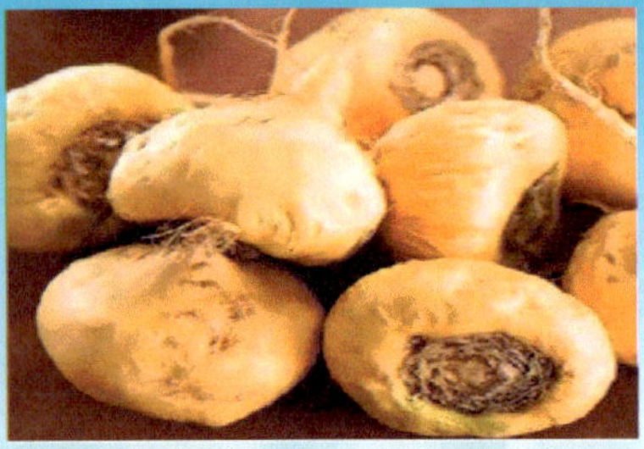

Maca Estrogen, energy, boost libido, mood improving, helps fertility.

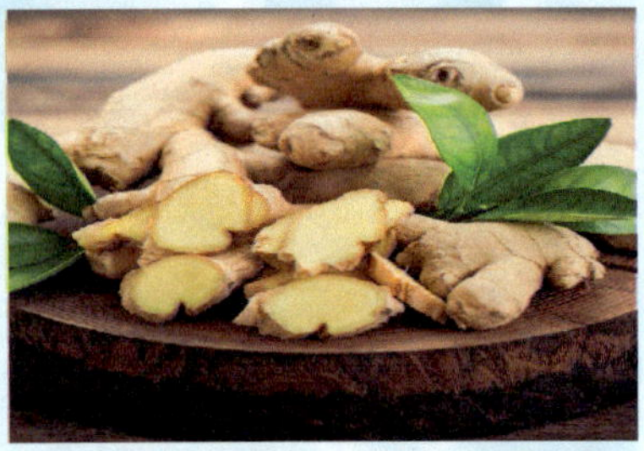

Ginger Prevents damage to DNA, help stress, gastrointestinal motility, nausea relief, arthritis inflammation, help infections heal faster.

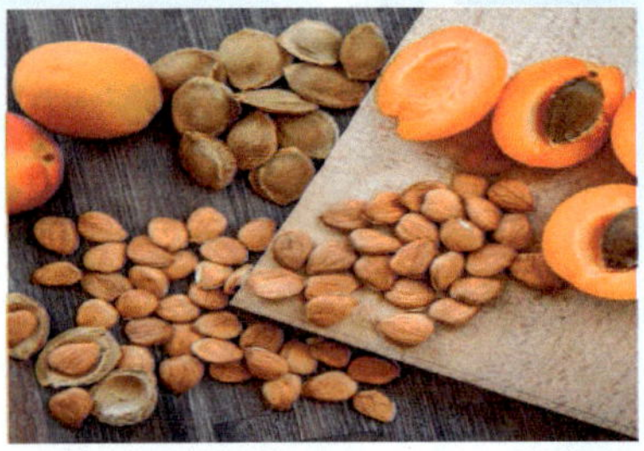

Apricot and seeds Cancer fighting, fiber, inflammation, lower blood pressure, arthritis, B17 Amygdalin, hair loss, digestive, gas bloating, thiamine, B1, lower blood pressure, heart health, omega 3, arthritis, zinc, liver health, immune defense, mood swings, increased resistance Alzheimer's disease, anti-aging.

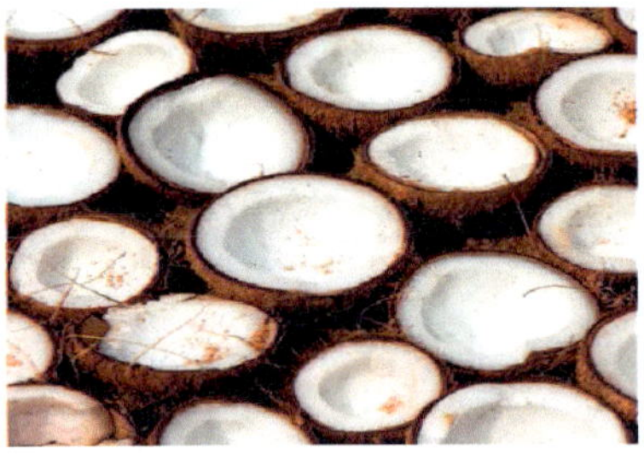

Coconut Control blood sugar, antioxidant, helps cancer fighting properties, kidney stones, amino acids, cytokines, heart health, blood pressure, fiber, supports bowels, digestive system, helps vitamin absorption, fights inflammation, brain function, skin, hair, helpful to remove parasites and worms.

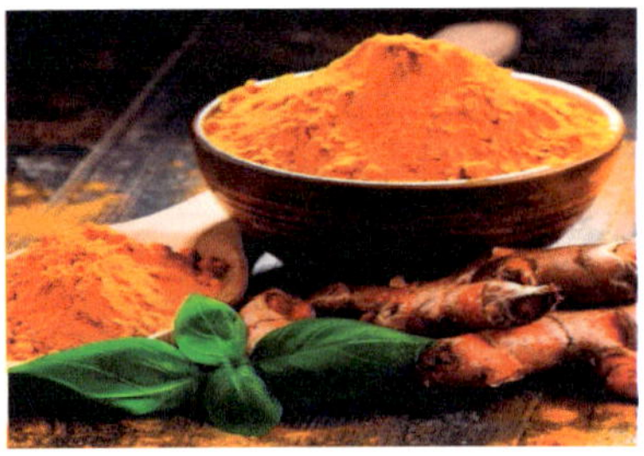

Turmeric Joint pain, immune booster, vitamin C, eye conditions, arthritis, hyperlipidemia, anxiety, muscle soreness, kidney health, skin disorders, respiratory infections, allergies, liver disease, depression, digestive system.

Food with Benefits and Superfoods

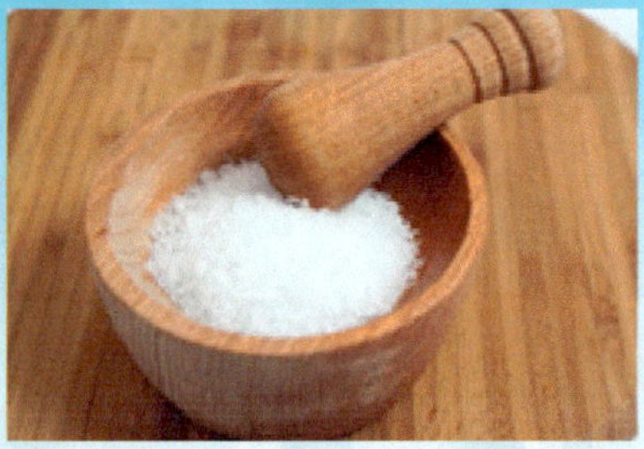

Salt recommendations Celtic salt, grey salt, Himalayan salt. Just a few grains of salt placed on the tongue and then drinking a glass of water will hydrate your body to the cell level well getting eight necessary trace vitamins daily.

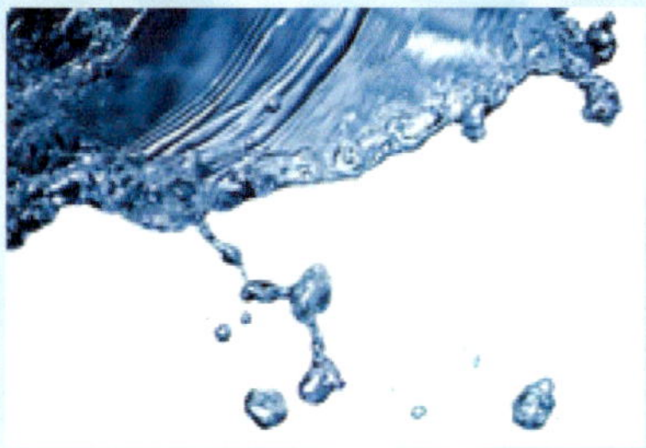

Water personally I rotate between Alkaline water and spring water. I feel as we age our gut health changes and I found that the alkaline water in better to balance our PH levels. I do not recommend alkaline water for anyone with kidney disease.

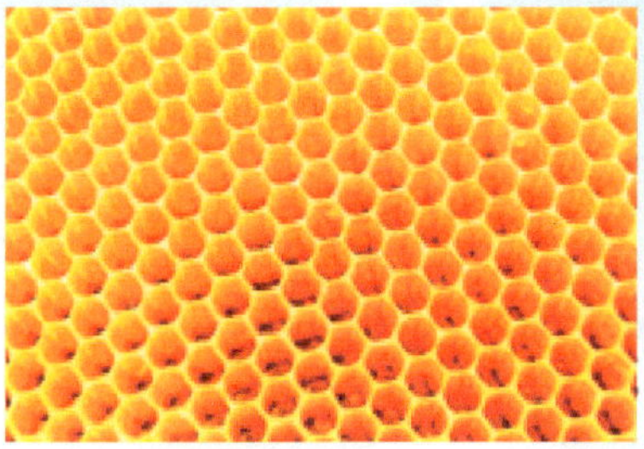

Honey is my favourite because this one product created in nature that is perfect in every way possible. Honey never expires like all other foods which is phenomenal! Health benefits include amino acids, iron, trace minerals, zinc, antioxidant, anti- inflammatory, anti-bacterial, helps nervous system, cardiovascular system, gastrointestinal, raw honey contains the most beneficial properties.

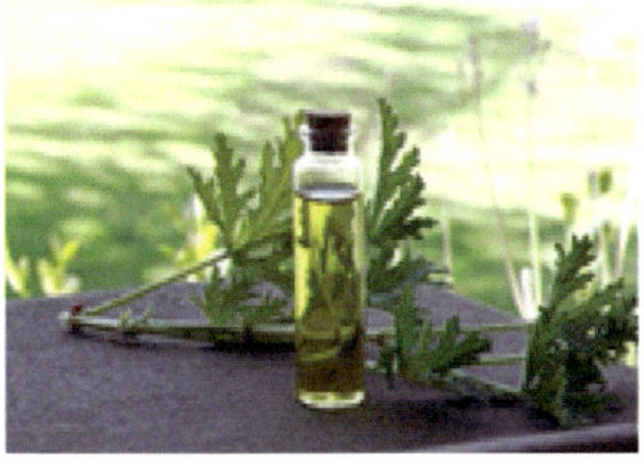

Oil recommendations Olive oil, Almond oil, Coconut oil, organic butter. When frying I try to use coconut oil because it has a higher smoke point which means it doesn't burn fast as the others. Allergy sufferers should stick with butter for frying on lower temperatures and olive oil on everything else. It Hydrate skin, hair, stretch marks, reduce puffy eyes (nut allergy people avoid).

Food with Benefits and Superfoods

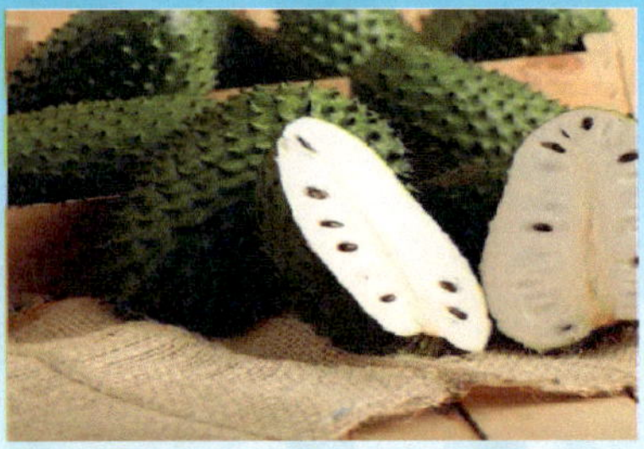

Soursop Cancer fighting, treats cystitis, diabetes, insomnia, headaches, hypertension, liver health, arthritic, anti-parasitic, anti-malarial, ulcers, vitamin C, protects skin from free radicals, digestion constipation, stabilizes blood pressure

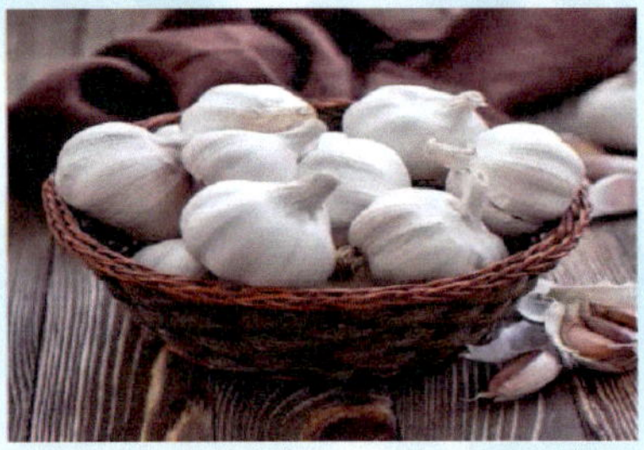

Garlic Medicinal properties, boost immune response, lower blood pressure, lowers cholesterol, reduces dementia, extend life, cancer prevention support, antibiotic, detox natural, reduces length of illness.

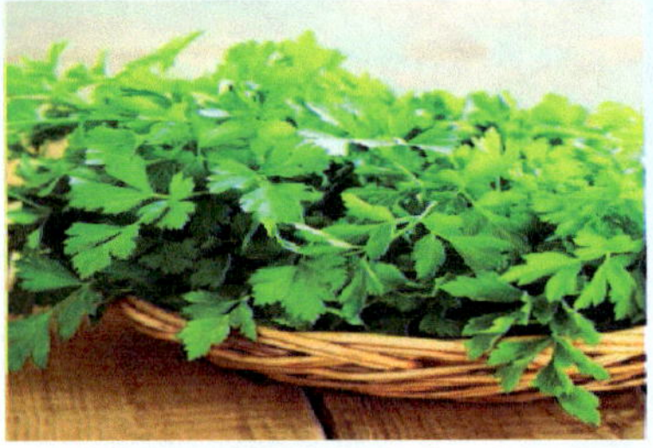

Parsley Detox, depression, antioxidants, bone health, gland health, diuretic effects, night blindness, lower cancer risk, immune system, heart health, ear health, Iron, helps arthritis, digestive support, gums, and teeth fresh.

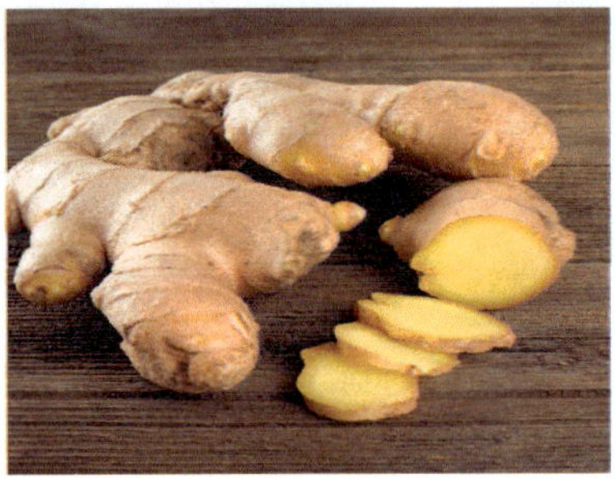

Ginger Magnesium, vitamin B6, C, Iron, fiber, pain in joints, digestive, inflammation, pain reliever, healing properties, gastrointestinal disorders, reduce nausea, weight loss, lowers cholesterol, protects nerve system, gut health, improves hormone levels and may increase fertility.

Seasonal Allergies

All my life I suffered with seasonal allergies, and someone mentioned trying one teaspoon of honey a day and explained to me that its process would take some time as all good natural products do but, do you believe that after sticking to this for six months which was easy cause I love honey, but it worked. I no longer suffer from seasonal allergies crazy good right!

The reason it works is the science behind it, the bee's collect pollen locally from flowers and weeds in your area that you experience your allergies from, therefore you receive trace pollen, and your body starts building up your immunity to those allergies.

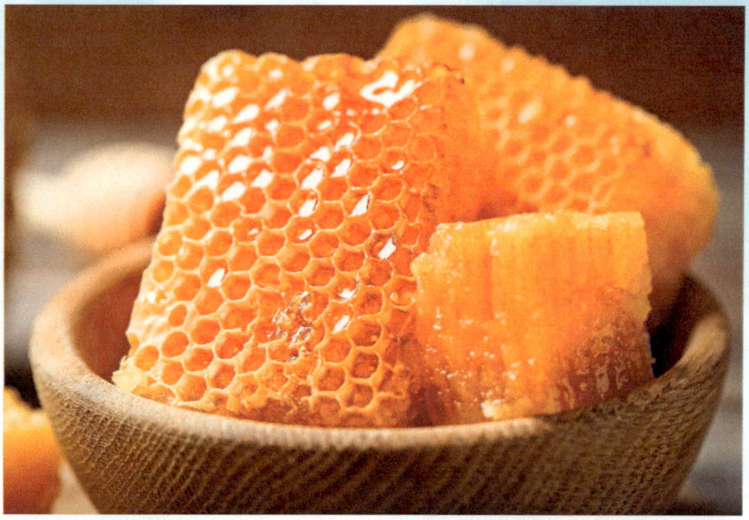

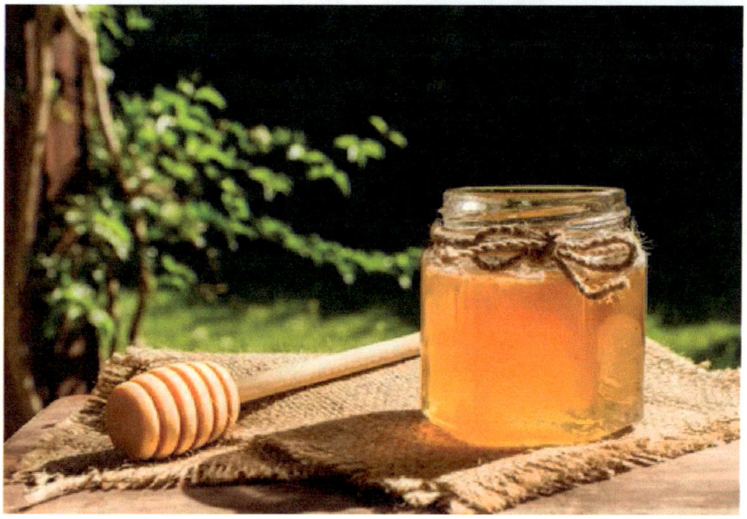

Natural Pain Relief

Did you know that the white willow tree bark is where a natural type aspirin comes from! Well, here you go take three-foot-long branches peel off the outer brown bark then chop or peel white inside bark into smaller piece this help release the salicin which has pain relieving properties as well as anti- inflammatory. At home, boil 4 cups of the mixture until it reduces to 2 cups. You can drink one cup of this for pain, its bitter so I add a little honey or cinnamon. In a pinch outside you can also chew the bark for pain relief, however it takes a bit longer to react possibly two hours this way.

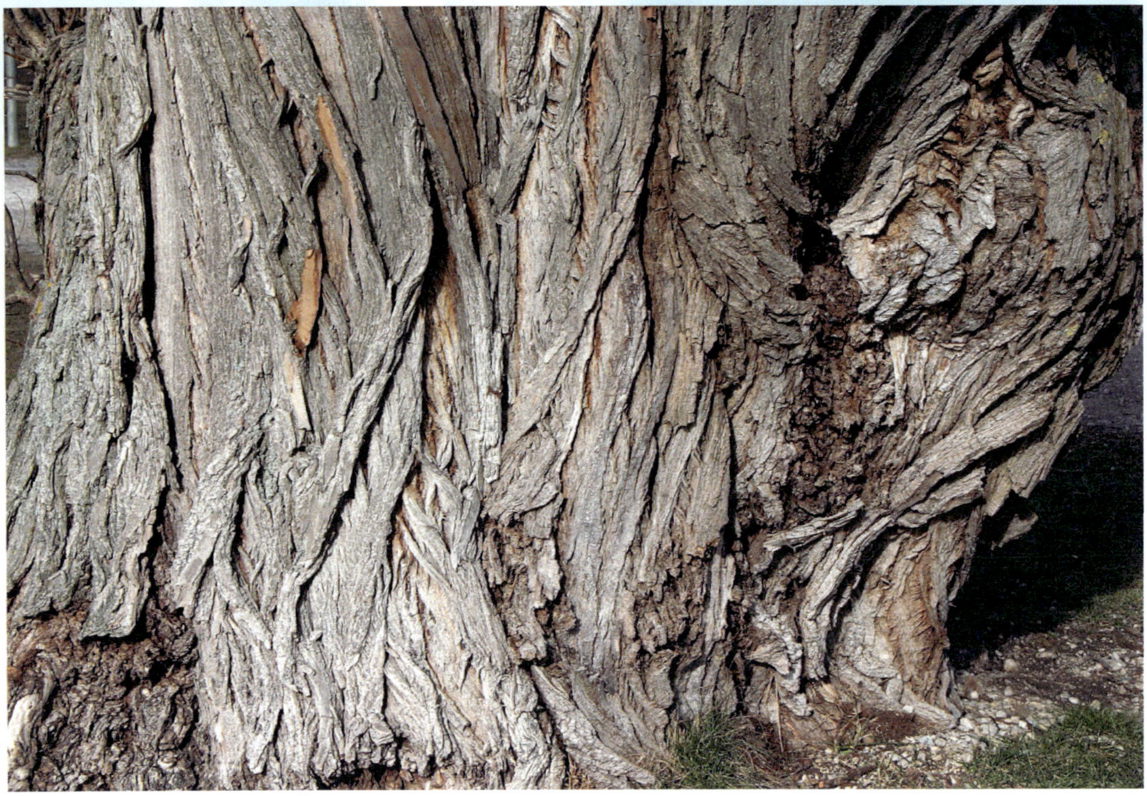

This is for your information only. Please seek doctor advice.

30 min chicken caprese

4 Boneless chicken breasts Extra virgin olive oil
Fresh garlic and basil
Salt and fresh ground pepper Fresh sliced mozzarella
Sweet Campari tomatoes (or tomatoes on hand) butter

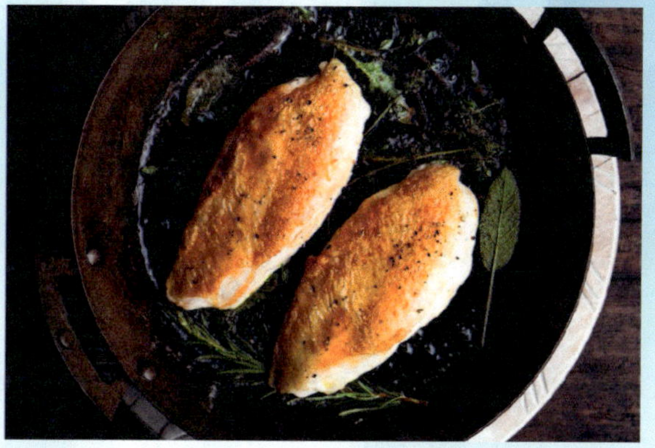

Instructions:

Add a pad of butter to pan and sear the chicken usually I slice the breasts in half to cook quicker!

Once seared add a drizzle of olive oil and turn to med heat add one cup of your tomato's.

Meanwell blend one clove garlic and bunch of basil with quarter cup of olive oil to make a paste.

Then add paste on top of each piece of chicken place one slice of mozzarella on each then lay a slice of tomato thin slice.

I usually place this type of chicken breast on a wonderful salad of greens. If you are ok with nuts toast some pine nuts and add for great nutty flavor

No pasta lasagna

Four or five large zucchini, one cup of flour, 3 eggs, crush tomato, coconut oil for frying zucchini, one cup parmigiano cheese, two cups mozzarella, salt, pepper

Ingredients:

Four to five generous size zucchini sliced long way thin as these will be your noodles. Once sliced get two bowls ready one with egg one with flour.

Flour first to dust them well then in egg then fry lightly watching until golden on each side. Remove onto a cloth or paper towel to absorb any extra oil.

Get your tray ready and cover the bottom with a little sauce regular tomato crushed. Crushed tomato cans 3 to 4 depending on how much sauce you like.

Then place your zucchini strips to cover bottom of the pan then a layer of sauce. Then a layer of mozzarella sprinkle of parmigiano cheese salt and pepper to taste Then add layers of sauce and repeat until you have two or three layers.

Top off with remaining sauce drizzle with olive oil bake 45 minute at 350F.

This is a vegetarian option, but you could add ground meat in-between the layers.

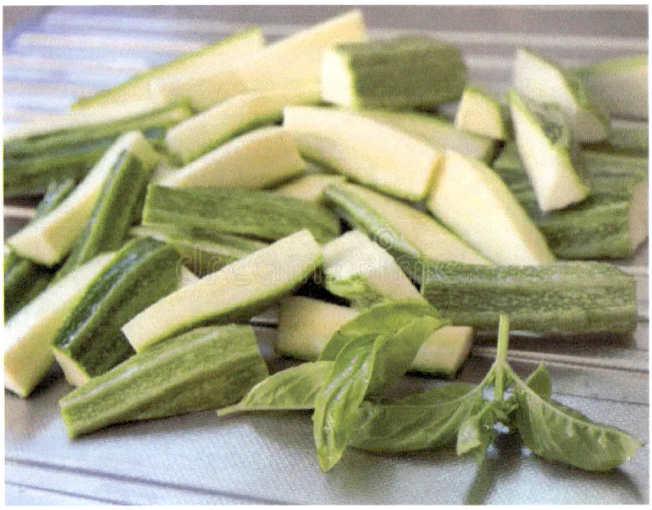

Stop buying gravy

Save the drippings from your roast turkey whole chicken by close to the last ten minutes of the cooking process you add two cups of water that you will add ½ teaspoon of salt ½ teaspoon garlic powder, ½ teaspoon of onion powder or sautéed onions, along with a quarter cup of butter or olive oil your choice.

After removing the meat pour the juice into and pot and bring to a boil. Well, that is boiling grab a mug and put ½ cup of flour in it then add slowly well stirring some boiling water just enough to make a thick runny paste stir until you remove any lumps. Then add this paste slowly well stirring to your boiling liquid and this will thicken your gravy. Add salt and pepper to taste.

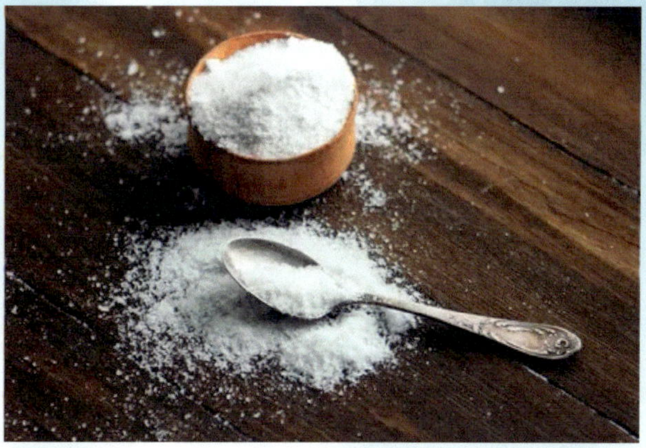

Ingredients:

Two cups of water, ½ teaspoon of salt, ½ garlic powder, ½ onion powder or 1/2 cup sauteed onions and 1 teaspoon minced garlic, quarter cup of butter or olive oil your choice.

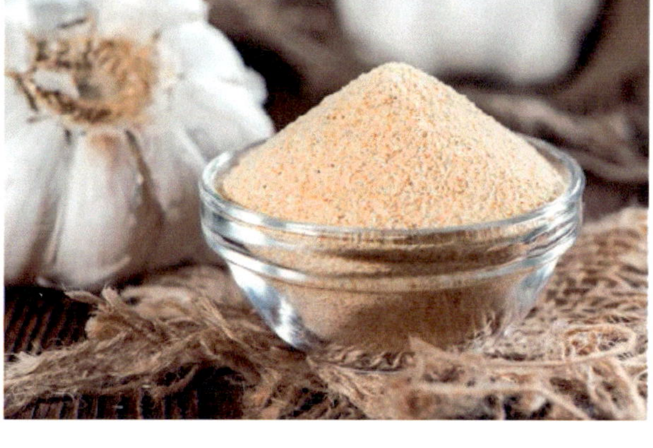

Winter salad

2 large cabbages shredded to which you add ½ cup of Himalayan salt, 5 cups of apple cider vinegar then add your veggies like chopped peppers, onion, garlic, carrots, celery, then your spices. I added caraway, mustard seed, coriander, cumin, black pepper, turmeric, cayenne, parsley, oregano, mint just a gracious sprinkling of each. Mix the entire ingredients well and then Pack in glass jars with rubber seal lids leaving little to no air. These will last in pantry for three months.

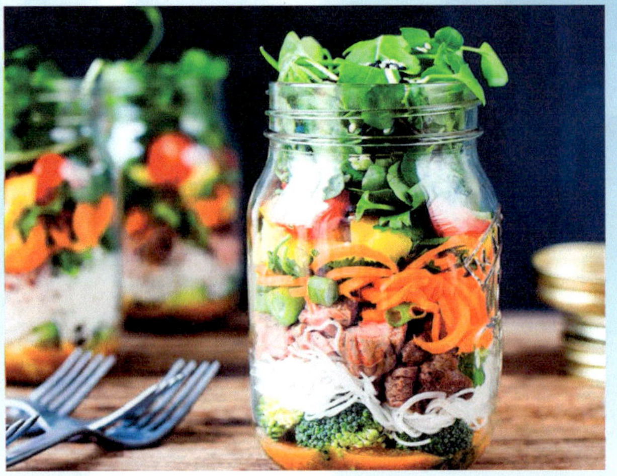

Baked dish with butternut squash

One butternut squash or any squash you like, ½ white onion, 1 large honey crisp apple or the apple you prefer, 1 sweet potato, 1 cup cherry tomatoes or any type of tomato on hand, 1 garlic clove, pinch of ginger, cover, or drizzle with two teaspoons of olive oil or butter organic or coconut oil. Bake at 350 for 35 minutes.

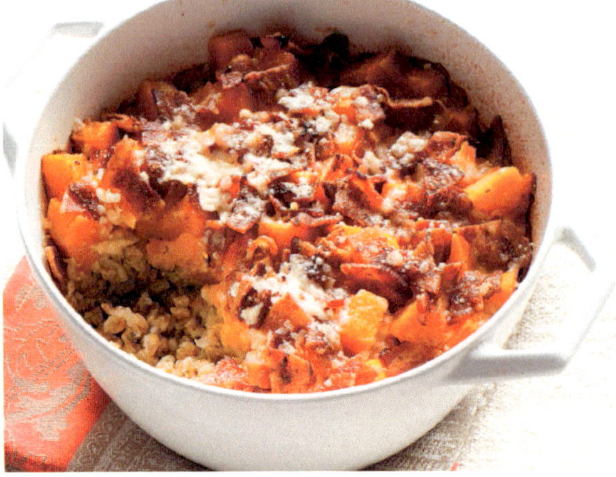

Bonus

Better then Botox for your skin

2cups rice any type 2cups flax seed

1 1/2 cups of water Aloe 1/3 cup

Castor oil 2 teaspoons Cheese cloth

Mix rice and flax seed in water in a saucepan, simmer on low heat for approximately 12 minutes. Let this cool lay your cheesecloth over a bowl pour rice mixture on top and then squeeze out liquid add the aloe stir then add the castor oil stir again pour into glass jar and seal. Good for 30 days in refrigerator.

Use all over skin topical only leave on for 15 mins and rinse off with icy water drying with cotton face towel for the softest skin ever naturally.

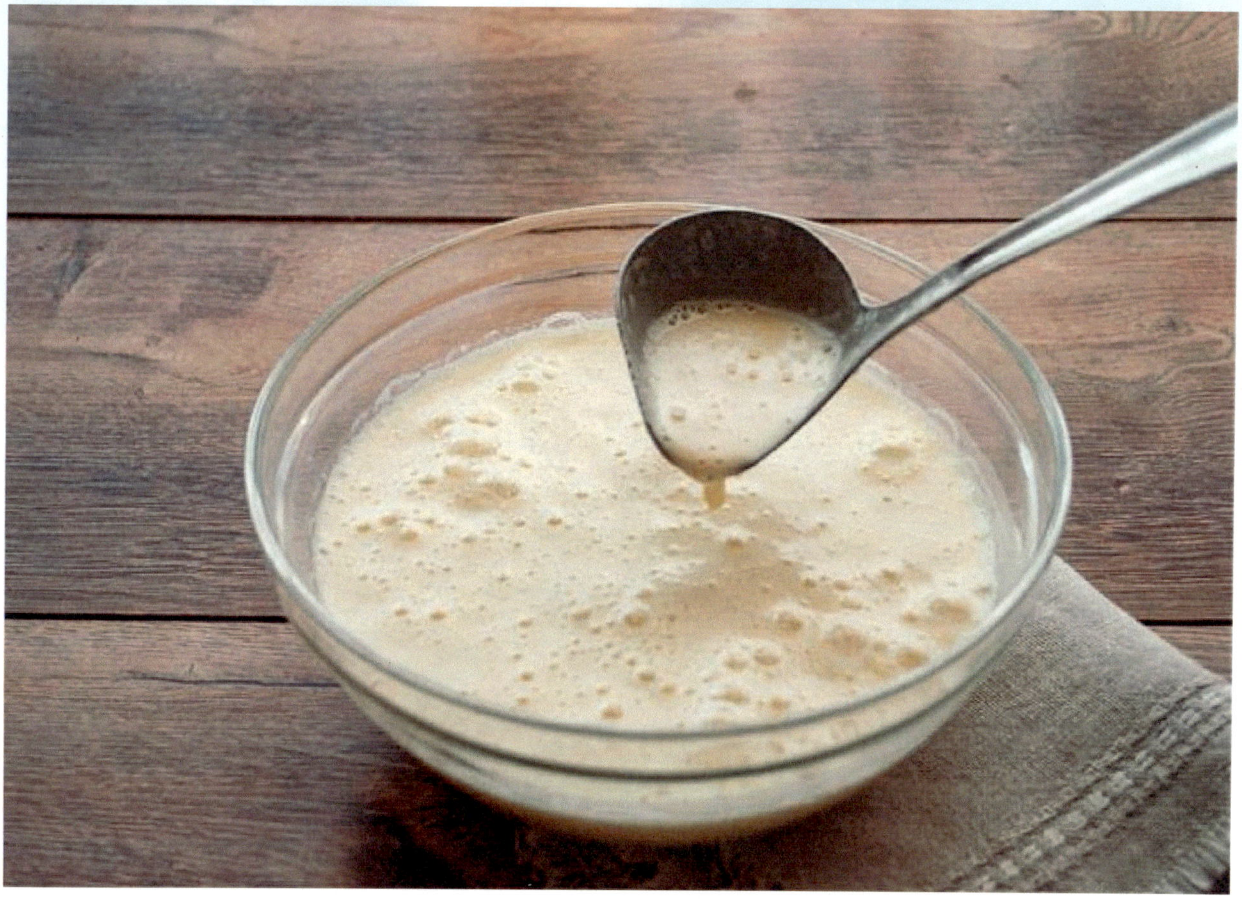

Conclusion

In conclusion, I want to express my heartfelt gratitude to each one of you who has embarked on this wellness journey with me. Your dedication to self-care and your commitment to better health are truly inspiring. Through stories shared in this book, I have shared my own struggles with bad eating habits and how am turning the clocks back by embracing whole foods, Today I can stand before you are feeling stronger healthy and vibrant than ever before.

I hope this will encourage you to continue prioritizing your well-being and caring deeply for yourself. Remember that you are worthy of the love and attention you pour onto others. Nurture your mind, soul, body, always striving for balance strength and embracing positive habits.

I would also like to extend my gratitude to those who have supported me and encourage me as well as those who have joined me along the way. Thank my family for the encouragement and feedback have been invaluable. Together, we have created a community that uplifts, motivates, and inspires one another.

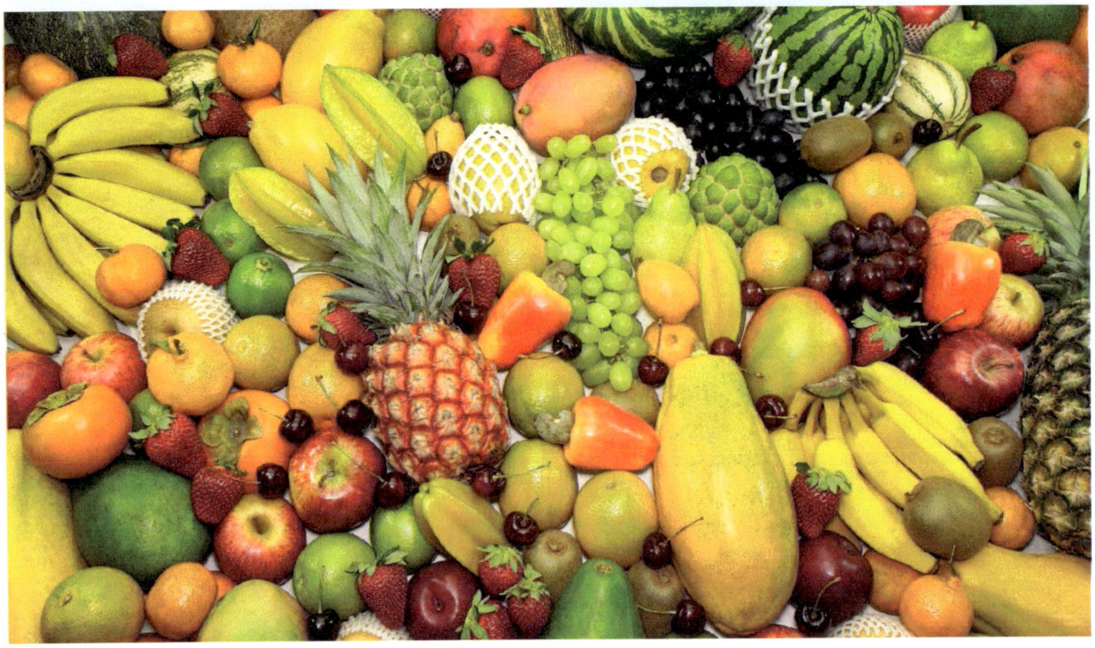

What Lies Ahead

Lastly, I invite you to keep a sharp eye out for my next book, where I will dive deeper into the world of wellness, meditation, sharing more stories, insights, and practical advice. Until then, may you continue to thrive, nourishing yourself with love, and spreading wellness wherever you go.

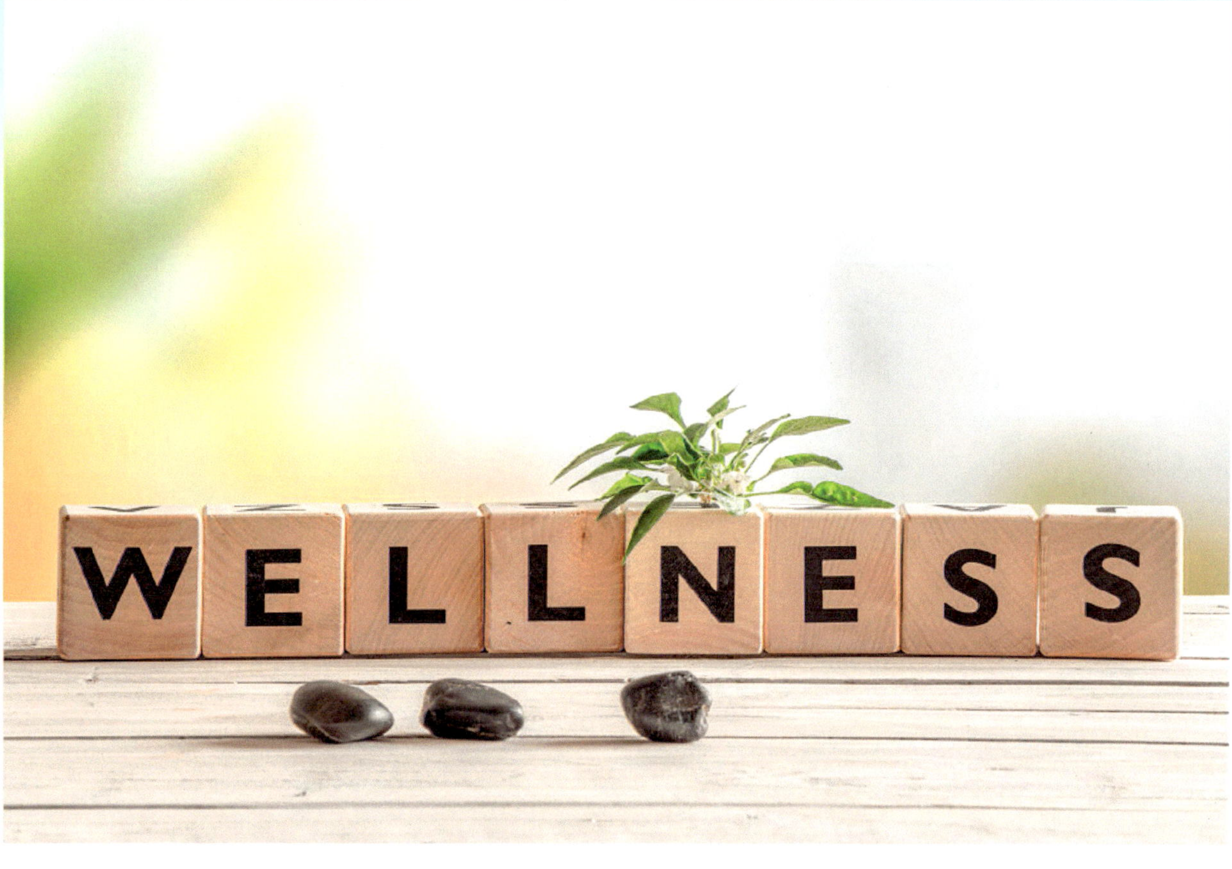

References

Some of the Remedies' ingredients can be bought from the given platform easily, my personal recommendations.

- Castor oil - holistic market Co. Amazon.
- Apricot seeds - Coyote - herbs Amazon.
- Sea moss - Renew active store Amazon.
- Celtic salt - organic original Celtic sea salt.
- Soursop tea - Ceylon flavours Amazon.
- Jojoba oil - Kanzy hair and beauty Amazon.
- Olive oil - first press - Colavita store Amazon.
- Pear soaps - local drugstore or Amazon.
- Mushrooms - The fantastic Fungi store Amazon.
- Honey Innisfil Creek - 6090 10th side road, Innisfil, Ontario
  LOL 1LO
  Contact No. 705-456-5093

Special Thanks to Eric Photographer

epicurevisuals@gmail.com

Made in the USA
Monee, IL
05 November 2026

67387143R00029